Fish, Faith, and Family

~

Ruth Schafer Lempert

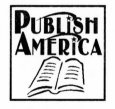

PublishAmerica
Baltimore

First printing

ISBN: 1-4241-9097-5
PUBLISHED BY PUBLISHAMERICA, LLLP
www.publishamerica.com
Baltimore

Printed in the United States of America

In memory of my daughter

Judith Ann (Lempert) Zaretsky

my parents

Sam Schafer and Kate (Oratz) Schafer

my sister

Esther (Schafer) Usdane

Schafer Family Tree

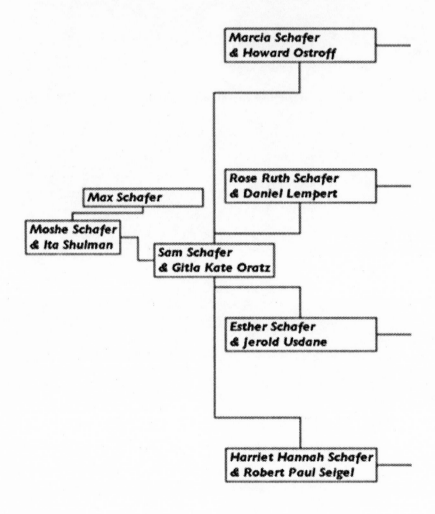

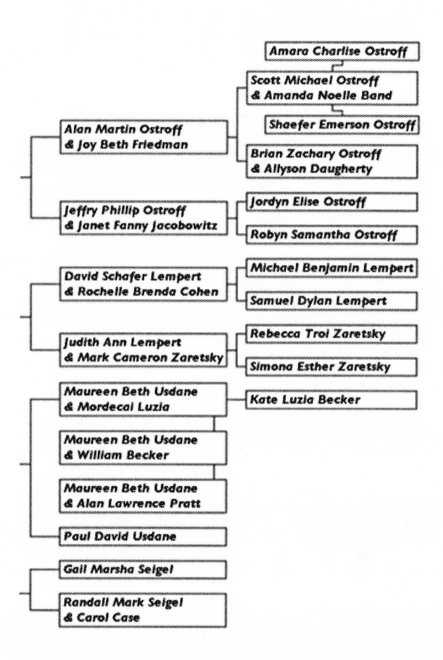

Amara Charlise Ostroff

Scott Michael Ostroff
& Amanda Noelle Band

Shaefer Emerson Ostroff

Brian Zachary Ostroff
& Allyson Daugherty

Alan Martin Ostroff
& Joy Beth Friedman

Jeffry Phillip Ostroff
& Janet Fanny Jacobowitz

Jordyn Elise Ostroff

Robyn Samantha Ostroff

David Schafer Lempert
& Rochelle Brenda Cohen

Michael Benjamin Lempert

Samuel Dylan Lempert

Judith Ann Lempert
& Mark Cameron Zaretsky

Rebecca Troi Zaretsky

Simona Esther Zaretsky

Maureen Beth Usdane
& Mordecai Luzia

Kate Luzia Becker

Maureen Beth Usdane
& William Becker

Maureen Beth Usdane
& Alan Lawrence Pratt

Paul David Usdane

Gail Marsha Seigel

Randall Mark Seigel
& Carol Case

Dedicated to my husband Daniel, my son David and his wife Shelley, my son-in-law Mark, to my sisters Marcia and Harriet, to my grandchildren Michael, Rebecca, Sam, and Simona, and to my nieces and nephews, Alan, Maureen, Jeffry, Paul, Gail, and Randy. They all encouraged me and personify and value the meaning of family.

And to all families who strive together to find their way through good times and bad, and to discover the meaning of family for themselves.

Acknowledgments

During the writing of this book I had help from many fine and patient people. Joyce Tavrow, childhood friend, was magnanimous with her time, sage advice, and unfailing encouragement. Heather Proctor proofread the draft and offered comments and suggestions. Roberta Baldo made criticisms that were helpful.

I appreciated the suggestions of my writing groups, and I wonder if I could have finished the book without them. My first writing group listened patiently while I read the work in progress. The second writing group listened over and over as I read from beginning to end. Camy Sorbello, my mentor, will always have my gratitude. We members of both writing groups originally met at Writers and Books when we took classes with Pat Bindert. I found Writers and Books, a literary organization in our city, to be a priceless resource. At the beginning of the writing of this book I had encouragement from my first teachers, Doug Stuber and Peter Marchand.

My father's life was greatly enhanced by the Association for the Blind (now called the Association for the Blind and Visually Impaired). They invariably gave him encouragement and support toward greater independence.

To all these family members, friends, and organizations, I am eternally grateful.

Table of Contents

CHAPTER ONE

Blind

They were like figures in a silent movie. We saw them standing on the other side of the emergency waiting room before they saw us. I could see Marcia crying. Harriet, was standing motionless next to her, pale and expressionless.

Esther and I walked faster. I ignored a tightening twist inside of me. Even before we reached them I called out, "What's the matter? What happened?"

"Dad was attacked and robbed in the store," Marcia managed to say between sobs. I already knew that. Esther had told me earlier when she called. She said the hospital people told her he'd be all right. They wouldn't tell her more. So why did my sisters look so stricken?

I asked again, "What happened?"

Swallowing hard, Marcia said, "A man came in the store and asked for money. Dad gave him 20 dollars and change. Maybe the robber was angry that there wasn't more. He choked Dad and left him for dead. Before he left he gouged out Dad's eyes. He's blind."

"He'll be blind the rest of his life." Harriet's voice was flat. She looked like a wooden statue with lips that moved.

Esther, silent since we entered the hospital, now spoke. "He's blind?" she asked, as though she did not understand the word. I didn't understand it either. Blind was other people, like Helen Keller. Blind was beggars in poor countries sitting on a street corner holding out a cup. I didn't know anyone who was blind. What did it mean to be blind?

"Who found him?" I needed to know, as though those details would help me make sense of this horror.

"The kid who lives upstairs came down to buy something, and found him lying on the floor," Harriet answered. "Dad was conscious by then, and the boy said that father whispered to him, 'Call an ambulance.'"

My mind recoiled as I tried to picture the scene. What if I had found him? What would I have seen? I averted my head as though I were looking at the violence I imagined. How could anyone gouge out someone's eyes?

The four of us sat in the emergency room stunned. I felt nothing. My mouth was dry, and I had a hard time talking. I kept wondering if a movie camera was recording everything I did. *This has got to be an awful movie I'm in,* I told myself. *This is not real.*

Just a few hours before the world had been normal. My main concern had been to read the Sunday morning paper. When Esther called to tell me he was in emergency, I was not alarmed—he'd been mugged before.

"Let's go pick him up," I had said. "He'll be ready to leave by the time we get there. I'll be at your house in a few minutes." She had looked somber, and I tried to allay her fears as she slid into the car. "Maybe he had to have a few stitches the way he did last year when a kid ran in and threw a can of peaches at him. Remember that redheaded teenager that pushed him down a couple of years ago? Dad broke his glasses when he fell, and that's what he complained about the most."

"I think it's worse this time," she said. How had she known?

Suddenly I stood up. "I have to see him," I said to my sisters. "I'll find out where he is." I left the waiting room to search for him, and found him in one of the emergency-room cubicles. His eyes and forehead were bandaged. There were bruises on his neck and face. He lay moaning and groaning, deep sounds of anguish or pain. He kept turning his head from side to side.

"Father, can I make you more comfortable?" He made no answer. He kept turning his head back and forth and moaning. How could I reach him? I tried to imagine how I would feel if someone had attacked me with such brutality. I would need to know I was safe. I took his large, rough hand in both of mine and I whispered, "You're safe now, Father. No one can hurt you. You're safe." I held his hand, hoping he could hear me.

My sisters found us, and we all sat around him talking softly. He must have known we were there because his moaning stopped, and he lay more quietly.

Harriet asked again, "Father, can I get you something?"

"A glass of water. My head hurts."

A nurse soon took him away to prepare for surgery. One of the doctors came to talk to us. "I'll clean the injury and see what we can do. Maybe we'll save some vision in the left eye."

By now each of us had called home, and more members of the family had arrived: our husbands and our children. As we sat, I kept futilely trying to grasp the reality of what was happening. I had never been touched by violence. I refused to read books or see movies or TV shows that were violent. I would not let it enter my life. As soon as Vietnam War scenes appeared on TV I turned it off. Brutality, murder—I kept them far away. How did they find me? I sat dry-eyed, waiting for the doctors to come back and say that my father would regain some vision and that we could go on as before.

After surgery the doctor gathered us together. His own eyes brimmed with tears. "I have never seen such a vicious injury inflicted on a person by another human being. Your father will be totally blind for the rest of his life. I'll tell him in a day or two. Will you be there with him for support?"

"We'll be there."

The family spent hours at the hospital, taking turns at meal times so we could help him. Actually, he preferred to help himself, asking only that we explain what was on his tray or requesting that we cut up his food. He began grumbling about the bandages that covered his eyes.

"When they gonna take off the bandages? I can't see what I'm doing."

We looked at each other in dread.

"The doctor will decide that, Father," one of us said.

Almost as soon as he could speak, my father asked in a hoarse voice, his throat still sore, "What about our trip?"

When my father was in the recovery room, I canceled the trip to Israel we had all been planning for over a year. How could he possibly undertake a strenuous journey in little more than a month? We had planned our family trip to begin on August 14, now only four and a half weeks away. "Travel is educational," our father had said, even when we had gone to see relatives in Utica, New York, a trip of about three and a half hours by car in those days. When he had suggested that the whole family take a trip to Israel we agreed, somewhat warily, that it might be exciting.

"We'll either have a wonderful time on a family trip, or we'll come back with one half not talking to the other half," I had said. With his encouragement we began pouring over brochures to find a trip that would not be too long or too expensive, one that would not move on the Sabbath from city to city, because he would not travel on the Sabbath. We had to coordinate vacation dates for all working members of the family, making sure that we would arrive back in time for school for the children.

We'd finally found a trip that met all our criteria. Our departure date had been set, and by the beginning of summer we bubbled with excitement. None of us had traveled much, and it would be the first airplane trip for some, including my father. The planning and preparation took many months, but the visit to the Holy Land had been my father's dream for over 50 years. When that robber walked into my father's store and robbed him of his sight, it appeared that he had also destroyed the fulfillment of a long-cherished dream. We needed to cancel the trip within the next few days or we would lose the whole deposit—a sizable amount. And he was subsidizing most of the trip. I felt responsible for salvaging as much as I could.

I looked at him lying in his hospital bed and answered his question. "I canceled the trip for now. We'll go when you're feeling better."

"You all go. I'll stay in a nursing home till you get back." The following day we talked about it again in his hospital room. We kept telling him we would go another year, while he kept insisting that we go without him.

His strength began to return rapidly. Although his voice was still raspy, the day after surgery he talked and joked with the nurses. On the second day after surgery his doctor spoke with me. "I think he's strong enough to hear the truth. Will you ask the family to meet me in his room tomorrow at three?"

How would my father respond when the doctor told him that he would never see again? What would he say or do? He had always been so active, unable to sit still for too long except in the synagogue. Even there, the service required standing up and sitting down every few minutes. He was impatient when we went someplace together, and he kept telling me to walk faster, to keep moving. I couldn't imagine him sitting quietly, waiting for someone to help him.

"What'll we do with the store?" Harriet asked. "Where should he live? There's so much to decide." She stopped, and then said, "I'm afraid."

In the days to come many acquaintances reading the frequent newspaper accounts of the story would ask, "Didn't you know how the neighborhood had changed?"

"Of course, we knew," I cried, "but he wouldn't listen to us." After a while I stopped defending the family. I needed to figure out how and why this had happened to us. Why was he still there when so many others had already left? He said later that his assailant had been "Big, strong, good-looking, maybe 30 years old. I never saw him before." It was no neighbor or customer. Twelve hours later an 18-year-old gas station attendant would be attacked in the same way and blinded.

The victims could never identify the perpetrator. No witness ever stepped forward. No one was ever charged with the crime.

My father had not been oblivious to the changes in the neighborhood, but he still cared for the avenue and the people who came in. For almost 50 years Sam Schafer and his fish market had served countless customers on Joseph Avenue. He had followed his philosophy of, "Keep the customer happy," and had enjoyed it so much that he gave no thought to retiring. During the last few years he had been mugged several times, and the family grew worried. We encouraged him to retire.

"Most people shop at supermarkets nowadays, Father," we said. "You can't be taking in much money. Does it pay to stay?" We carried on this conversation fairly often—a few times a month.

One day I made him sit down and listen to me. "Look, Father," I explained, "the neighborhood is dangerous now. Get out and sell the store and the whole building."

"My neighbors like me. They wouldn't hurt me."

"It doesn't matter whether your neighbors like you. Strangers move in and out all the time," I answered. "They're dealing in drugs, gambling, prostitution, and who knows what else? Everyone who can moves out as fast as possible. There's violence all around. Most of your neighbors are stuck here. You don't have to stay."

My father turned away, and then he looked back at me. "What would I do all day if I stopped working?" he asked. I didn't know how to answer. I said no more.

At 72 he was almost as strong as all four of his sons-in -law put together, although they were practically half his age. Barely five feet four inches tall, he was stocky and muscular. For decades he had hauled big wooden boxes of fish bedded in ice, lifted cases of groceries and soda water, lugged huge barrels of herring, smoked fish, or pickles from the walk-in cooler at the back of the store to the sidewalk in front. He enjoyed talking to his customers, exchanging pleasantries, and discussing local news or world events. Meeting different people every day, talking to them about their problems—those were the things he relished.

He had never taken a vacation. The store was always open except for the Sabbath and the Jewish holidays. Outside of work, only his family and his religion were worthy of his time. A few months earlier my sisters and I were together discussing what to do. Esther said, "He's not going to retire. I'll ask Jerry to help him look for a place to relocate." Jerry, Esther's husband, was our wheeler and dealer.

"That's a great idea," I said.

"Good luck to Jerry," said Marcia.

"Tell him there's a store for sale on Monroe Avenue," added Harriet.

Everyone was in favor of this plan. A flurry of activity followed as they searched for a new location. Jerry announced soon afterward, "Your father and I found a place on Monroe Avenue. He's going to make a purchase offer." The purchase offer was made, but the deal fell through. The flurry stopped. Why hadn't we kept on looking? Guilt, like a horde of black flies, would come back to plague us over and over.

Even my father would one day say to me, "Why didn't you tell me to leave?"

"I did, Father," I answered gently. "We all did, but you wouldn't listen."

"You should have told me again and again. I would listen."

But he did not say that until months later. Right now we had to think about tomorrow, about revealing his future to him, telling him the truth about his blindness. The neighbors who liked him and would never hurt him had not been able to protect him from the forces of mindless savagery.

CHAPTER TWO

Response

As we crowded into my father's hospital room, I pushed my way to his bedside and grabbed his hand in greeting. He circled my wrist with his thumb and forefinger and said, "Your arm is too skinny." Paul, Esther's son, put a hard candy in his grandfather's hand. He knew it was a favorite treat. I looked at everyone quickly and then stared at the floor. This was going to be hard. I didn't know what anyone would say. What words could any of us use to make it easier?

I had perfected a technique that protected me from pain. I imagined wrapping each organ in my body carefully in impermeable insulation. Not even a sharp little stab could get though that insulation. In this way I was not numb, but I protected myself against a flood of emotions too strong to bear.

I felt well wrapped when the doctor came in and began talking to my father. He was kind, but matter of fact. "Sam, the injury to your eyes was extremely severe. There was nothing we could do to repair the damage. You are blind, and we can't do anything to bring your vision back." The doctor stopped, and we all sat waiting for my father's response.

At first he said nothing. We waited. I kept looking at the floor as though an unusual animal lay there. *Is it easier to be born blind or to suddenly have the world turn black?* I wondered. *Is the world really black if you can't see, or are there colors whirling about in front of you?* Perhaps it is better to lose your sight slowly. You have time to get used to the idea. Was it harder to adjust if you were older? Gone would be my father's visual observations of the people around him, of how he looked at a party, if he had ketchup on his jacket, if other people were smiling or frowning. Gone was his option to drive a car, to remain completely independent.

How could my father survive this? We waited for him to break the silence. "I guess I'll have to learn to live with it," he finally said calmly.

We all began talking at once, telling him how we would help him. "I'll be your secretary, Father," I said, "and your chauffeur."

Everyone offered to run errands, shop, take him to the barbershop. Each of us proposed that he come to live with us. His grandsons told him they would help all they could. Much later he confessed that when the doctor had finished speaking, he thought for one brief and awful instant that he would go mad, but no one in that room guessed the turmoil within him. In the 20 years of his blindness he rarely spoke of the loss of his eyes. After a few years he said more than once, "Your sight is a precious gift." His vocabulary had not contained the word "precious," nor had he talked of gifts. Somewhere he had learned that phrase, and when he said, "Your sight is a precious gift," his voice had a catch, and then he was silent. I knew it was one of those times when his grief overcame him.

But that first night when he knew of his blindness, he didn't seem to believe what the doctor told him. "I think I see something," he exclaimed. "Isn't that the window over there?" He pointed to the blank wall.

"No, it's not there, Father." Several times he excitedly pointed to something he "saw." Each time he expressed disappointment when I told him he was mistaken.

Do people who lose their sight suddenly still think they see things? I thought of patients who have phantom pain in a limb they have lost. Maybe this illusion of seeing things is the same idea—a denial of the grief of losing a part of yourself forever.

* * *

The story of the savage attack on my father and his undaunted response were front-page news in our local paper and in papers everywhere. Cards and letters began pouring in from all over the world. We sat at his bedside in the hospital, reading every single message to him, marveling at all the people he knew who took the time to send words of encouragement. We marveled even more at the complete strangers who sent cards and notes. One morning I read a message to him from a group of nuns who said prayers for him in Rome. Knowing what an observant Jew he was, I wondered about his response. He smiled and said, "I need all the prayers I can get." Another time I heard him mutter to himself, "Maybe it will all be interesant." (interesting)

The question of our family trip was still unresolved. As my father lay in the hospital recovering from his injuries, we remained at an impasse. He insisted that we go without him, and we were firm in our resolve to wait until he could go with us. He loved his adopted country fiercely, but he had always wanted to visit the Holy Land, to see the sacred places of the Old Testament, and to tread on the hallowed earth where Abraham, Isaac, and Jacob had walked. He kept telling us what a burden it would be to have a blind person along on the trip. "I'll always need someone with me," he reminded us. When he saw that we were adamant in our resolve to go together or not at all, he finally said, "All right, I'm going." We looked at him in astonishment.

"I'll ask the doctor, " I said.

"If your father wants to go to Israel he should be able to go by your departure date," the doctor said.

Quickly I called Sylvia, our travel agent. "The trip's on again," I crowed.

"I'm not surprised," she said. Pleased as she was, Sylvia needed permission from the tour company to accept a blind person. She obtained permission the same day, after explaining to the tour director that my father had seventeen members of his family along to assist him. I had not realized how few people with disabilities traveled and how reluctant and unsure travel companies felt about having them.

While he was in the hospital one or more of us came every day to help, although he insisted on doing everything himself. At dinnertime he only wanted to know what was on his plate. We offered to cut up his food to make it easier for him, but we stopped that when we met Mrs. Carley.

The night before his release from the hospital, July 13th, Mrs. Carley, a representative from the Association for the Blind, arranged to speak to the family. A large room had been reserved for our meeting. She would explain how to help our father adjust. She brought with her a wealth of paraphernalia—a talking clock, a Braille watch, a guide stick, and many other implements to aid a sightless person. All were laid out on a table. We sat on hard folding chairs, tired and disheartened. Mrs. Carley stood before us, explaining the harm of being overprotective and reiterating how important it was to allow my father to do things on his own. My father seemed to know this already; he discouraged well-meaning but over solicitous attention.

"I'll be coming to your house to help you in your new life, Sam," Mrs. Carley told him. "Don't forget," he answered.

That night in the hospital she told us, "Life will be different, but that doesn't mean your father can't do many of the activities he enjoys." She made it sound as if so much were possible. Listening to her and seeing the table covered with aids for the blind, I finally grasped the reality of what had happened, and there in that room, I cried for my father for the first time.

He left the hospital on the Friday after the attack. Harriet, a nurse at Strong Memorial Hospital, was our own family health professional upon whom we relied for all things related to sickness, treatment, and recovery. She insisted he rest when he came home. Because it was the beginning of the Sabbath, he would naturally rest anyway. He told Harriet he could walk to services Saturday morning. On the Sabbath he did not drive nor allow himself to be driven. Although bandages still covered his eyes and his forehead, we could not dissuade him. Harriet reminded him it was not yet a full week since the attack, and he was still recovering.

"Father, you don't have all your strength back. It might be smart to take it easy and rest for a few days."

"I'm tip top. You can rest. I just need one person to go with me. Lemme call one of the boys." Ignoring Harriet's advice, he made plans to attend Sabbath services the next morning. Worries assailed us. Was he strong enough to walk the two miles? This was his first venture into the world since his "accident," as we sometimes referred to the savage attack. Would it pose great emotional stress so soon after his ordeal? During our discussions, David, my 15-year-old son, volunteered to go to services with him that morning and sit with him in the men's section. I went, too, although I could not sit with him because Beth Sholom was Orthodox. I sat with the women.

My father was always among the first to arrive at services, but this Saturday we started our walk a little later. With coaching from Harriet, he got up and dressed himself and took his cold breakfast. Holding David's arm, he walked two miles to shul. Neither one of them spoke about the previous Sunday nor referred to it. They talked about the hot July weather, about the morning traffic near Cobb's Hill that my father could hear, traffic that he had watched countless times before. It was as though he were making the walk for the first time. He listened more closely to the sounds—the voices around him, the flow of cars, the heavy lumbering noise of buses passing by. Had he paid attention to the appearance of the street before? Had it ever been important to notice how wide the street was as he crossed it? How high was the curb at the other side? How busy did the intersection sound? Was it uphill or downhill at Highland Avenue? He knew this area well, but now he took on a new relationship with the street.

My father and David entered the Temple hallway. Because the service had been in progress for about an hour—late for my father, who usually was there at the very beginning—there were few people outside of the sanctuary. David described how he felt and what happened.

"We walked through the hallway toward the sanctuary where the doors were closed. I could hear the low hum of people praying. Maybe some of them were asking for good health, or a better job or for peace in the world. I had a feeling that our entrance into the sanctuary might

24

cause a stir. Grandpa's picture had been in the paper all week. His progress in the hospital was news every day. I knew he was well known at the temple, and I thought some of his friends might crowd around him, and we wouldn't be able to get to our seats. And I knew no one would expect him to be back at services so soon. So we got ready to go in. Grandpa was wearing dark glasses over the long bandages that covered his eyes. He held his head up and took a deep breath. I thought he was breathing in whatever courage he could find in the air around him.

"I opened the door to the sanctuary, and the two of us walked in. No one seemed to notice us at first. People kept praying and talking, but then, all at once there wasn't a sound—like a cloud of silence dropped over the room. I felt that everyone there was watching us as we walked to our seats. I felt proud that I was with a man of such strength and faith—that even though he was attacked a few days before, he would not miss a Sabbath service. We kept walking to our seats in the silence, never stopping, even though a small crowd started to follow us. These were his fellow worshippers. He had seen them every day for years. Now he would never see them again. They were glad to have him back. One man said, 'It's good to see you here, Sam.'

"Grandpa started to say, 'It's good to see,' but he corrected himself in mid-sentence. 'It's good to hear your voice,' he answered. I felt so proud to stand with my grandfather, but I was fifteen, and I couldn't figure out why the God that Grandpa trusted all his life and that he had faith in would let something like this happen."

From the balcony I saw David and my father when they entered the sanctuary. I was not prepared for the hot, quick tears that blurred my eyes as they came into view. David walked tall. My father, with his bandaged eyes, held David's arm above the elbow, the way he was to hold everyone who would lead him from then on. When they sat down and found their place in the prayer book, the service resumed.

In our discussions of where our father would live, we all agreed that his own house would not do. We understood that blind people can live independently and alone, but we were reluctant for our father, at 72 years of age, to begin his blind life alone. Before my father left the hospital, we met with the social worker to discuss his living arrangements. Each of us volunteered to take him home. He had never wanted to live with any of his children, but when he left the hospital he agreed to move in with Harriet, his "baby." All of us, including Harriet, thought it would be temporary. Some of his wounds required treatment and bandaging. With her nursing skills, Harriet's home seemed the best choice for his recovery.

I thought he could come to stay with me for several months, and possibly we could take turns having him. We knew so little of what it means for a blind person to become accustomed to a place. It took him months to find his way around Harriet's house. We saw that moving my father from one place to another would be extremely difficult for him. Without too much said by any of us, Harriet's home became his permanent home. He would often say, "I could never have made it without her." We all knew that to be true. Eight-year-old Randy, Bob and Harriet's son, became his grandfather's roommate for several years until another room was constructed. Harriet's husband, Bob, gave his support and help in every way. Eleven-year-old Gail played checkers with him, a game he had always enjoyed. (They used a special set for the blind) Frequently she walked to the bank around the corner with him. When he needed someone to look up a phone number he would ask Gail.

No sooner was my father settled into his new home than my father along with the rest of us, began preparing for the trip. With less than one month to go, he learned to use the guide stick to get from place to place. From Mrs. Carley he learned little tricks to help him get his bearings. She taught him to eat neatly, explaining that in restaurants all over the world, food is arranged in a certain pattern. He mastered that pattern. He learned to use the dial telephone—the kind most of us had then. A piece of tape was put on the dial at the number five. Feeling the tape, he figured out where the other numbers were. He could dial as fast and as accurately as anyone. Because he still had a good memory, he remembered a long list of phone numbers and could make most of his own calls unassisted.

During those first weeks of his blindness, we all helped him master new skills. We were also busy finding someone to buy or rent the store, selling out the merchandise in the store, and organizing the last-minute details of the trip. At the same time my husband, children, and I were also preparing to move into a new home. We had no time to shop for clothes for the trip, and I noticed in our pictures and slides afterward, that I wore the same clothes day after day. We were exhausted before we left, yet buoyed by the anticipation of our pilgrimage. So ready or not, on August 14 we left the United States—all eighteen of us.

Because the attack on my father had received a great deal of news coverage, we found once we began traveling that reporters awaited us at every airport. My father was gracious and affable to all of them. He enjoyed answering their questions. In fact, when no one met us at Arad, a new development town, my father asked in a disappointed voice, "Don't they know we're here?" Wherever we went, people paused to look at us. And why not? We were a motley group, ranging in age from eight to 72. We all looked somewhat haggard, yet we must have exuded an emotion that combined pleasure, pain, and surprise that we were on our journey after all—a journey that most of us had been almost certain would never take place.

The tenor of the trip was set early in the tour. At one of the first sites we visited, there were a number of steps and loose stones strewn about from ongoing excavation. The footing appeared precarious, and our guide suggested that my father might prefer to wait in the bus while we explored. When we told my father what the guide had suggested, he thought a moment. Rather tartly he replied, "I didn't come all this way to sit in the bus while everyone else sees the country." That was the last time we asked if he wanted to sit in the bus. If he felt tired or if the going got rough, he would tell us.

In our effort to see as much as possible, we had jammed too much into each day. We were up early each morning and adhered to an ambitious schedule of sight-seeing that kept us moving all day and into the evening. My father kept up with us and was, indeed, rather impatient with those who complained of being tired. "Let's keep moving," he said, raising his voice so the laggards trailing behind would be encouraged to quicken their pace.

I said, only half in jest, "You should be traveling with a younger crowd."

CHAPTER THREE

Trip

We established a pattern on this trip that we would follow on subsequent family trips. The grandsons took turns sharing a room with their grandfather. Only Randy, his year-round roommate, knew what to expect. All the grandsons except Alan rotated nights. Alan, Marcia's son, had been married in June, and the trip was our wedding present to him and his bride. My father was a sound sleeper. It did not disturb him if the boys came in at odd hours of the night. He did not want to wake anyone up to help him find the bathroom. Nevertheless, he sometimes would wake his roommate by bumping his way through the room with his guide stick. Paul, Esther's son, described a typical night.

"I'd be sleeping in my bed, and I'd hear a crinkling sound. It would get louder and louder. I'd look over, and I'd see his hand in a bag of hard candy. Each piece of candy was wrapped in cellophane, and he was trying to unwrap them. I'd hear crinkling and crinkling and crinkling and crinkling. I didn't get mad because it was Grampa, but if anybody else had been crinkling, I would have been really angry. Sometimes he would shave in the middle of the night. He'd probably felt his face. If it felt rough to him, he'd hoist himself out of bed and head for the bathroom. He always told us, 'There's no time like the present.' The rooms were small, but it would take Grampa a long time to get to the bathroom. Sometimes he bumped into a wall. His guide stick would clack and bang against the furniture and walls. So with all the crinkling and banging, clacking and bumping, and the razor buzzing on and off, it was hard to get to sleep again."

One night when it was my son, David's turn, he was awakened by my father's screaming and yelling in his sleep. David was able to calm and reassure him. "You're safe, Grandpa, you're safe," he said. "It's just a bad dream you're having."

At every hotel on our trip, we wanted to find the room easiest for my father to move around in. The best room was always the one in which he could find his way to the bathroom unassisted. The teacher from the Association for the Blind had taught us that in every bedroom, the bed should be next to or very near the wall, and furniture should be arranged to serve as a guide to the bathroom. Bearing this in mind, we always found at least one room from among those assigned, in which the bed was in the right place, and we could arrange the tables and chairs. My father could get up from his bed, find the wall as one of us would instruct him, and use the tables and chairs we had arranged to enable him to reach his destination. This meant, of course, that we did some changing of assigned rooms.

My sisters and I allowed time to work with our father immediately after our arrival in a new setting so he would feel as independent as possible in each hotel. A room in which it was easy for him to learn getting around took twenty or thirty minutes of orientation. We showed our children how to work with their grandfather, too, so that at any given point there would always be someone available to help.

Our sightseeing continued at a dizzying pace. The Western Wall in Jerusalem is a portion of the ancient Temple of Solomon, destroyed by the Romans in the year 70. Here religious services are held, and we all prayed there, men on one side, women on the other. My father touched the Wall as Alan, Marcia's son, described this most sacred of places.

"Do you feel the big blocks of stone? Let me put your hand in the crack between these huge blocks, Grandpa. Do you feel the pieces of paper?"

He told my father about all the little pieces of paper that were stuffed in the cracks between the massive blocks of stone that made up the

Wall. On each piece of paper was a prayer or a fervent request that many supplicants left.

At the Dead Sea, we all swam in the heavy, oily-feeling water. The sea is so full of salt that it is impossible to sink. My father enjoyed splashing about in the water with us. He had also heard that the Dead Sea had healing powers, and we knew he was hoping it could help restore his vision. He splashed about, ducking his face in the water. If he felt disappointment at the lack of change in his vision, he did not show it. A sharp stab of sorrow sliced through me as I watched him, knowing how he kept hoping his sight would return. We all felt his disappointment

We spent a weekend at a kibbutz, a commune in which labor, child rearing, and most other tasks were shared by the Israelis who chose to be in it. Every kibbutz had a main purpose, such as agriculture, handwork or arts, etc. Kfar Giladi, a mountain resort kibbutz, was cool and refreshing after the heat of the desert. We arrived at the kibbutz shortly before sundown on a Friday and immediately began running from room to room, trying to find the best room for my father. We knew he would not do any moving once the Sabbath started. We must have looked like a scene from a Keystone Cops movie, dashing about with our suitcases, darting in and out of rooms.

"I think I've got a good room for Grandpa," Maureen, Esther's 17-year-old daughter might call out.

"Ours is better. The bed is only a couple of feet from the bathroom. Take a look," Judy, my daughter who roomed with Gail might answer.

My father wanted to attend Sabbath services on the Friday we arrived at the kibbutz, but the caretaker of the little synagogue there did not think he could muster up the ten men on such short notice. My father rounded up his grandsons and sons-in-law. Counting himself, that made nine. The caretaker was the tenth man—now they had a minyan. Services were conducted on the kibbutz for the first time in many months.

At Jericho, a reporter and photographer from the *Jerusalem Post* met us to interview my father. I had not imagined that so many who had read about the attack wanted to know how my father was managing on the trip and how he was enjoying it. After a lengthy question-and-answer session, which my father thoroughly relished, the photographer attempted to take some pictures with his expensive camera. For some reason, it jammed and could not be used.

The frustrated photographer was very upset. He was too far from any other place where he could get the necessary equipment. Looking at my husband, Dan, who was holding our own little Kodak Instamatic, the photographer asked, "Can I borrow your camera?" Reluctantly, Dan took out our film, and gave the photographer a new roll. The photographer took a number of pictures, and the next day there was a great shot in the *Jerusalem Post* of my father with Esther descending the stone steps in Jericho.

So we traveled the length and breadth of Israel, walking through the bazaars of Arab Jerusalem, climbing the steps of the mosques (which my father would not enter because he did not feel it appropriate for an observant Jew to enter a house of worship of another faith), ascending Masada in a cable car. At the president's invitation, we visited his house and had a special audience with his secretary and a tour of the presidential house.

My father saw everything through our eyes. We described the sky, the flowers, the green of the shrubs and trees, the mixture of cultures and people. He listened to the babble of tongues spoken throughout the land. He smelled the bougainvillea, the foods prepared in the kiosks of the streets, touched the Tomb of the Patriarchs. I described the camel caravan we saw—a Bedouin silhouetted against the desert horizon while a silvery plane flew overhead. It was a land of such contrasts, so old and so new.

We returned home in late August. Everyone returned to work, to school, or to a regular routine. For my father, it meant learning to live every day as a blind man.

CHAPTER FOUR

Reinvention

My father never had hobbies or leisure activities, nor had he ever taken a vacation. His family, his work, and his religion occupied every moment of his life. Now he began to pursue new interests and activities with a zest and enthusiasm that amazed us, while at the same time he relearned tasks that once had been simple for him. With Harriet's expert coaching, he once again made his own breakfast, washed dishes, peeled potatoes, changed sheets, and asked for more to do. He began listening to talking books.

"You ought to start reading books. You can learn so much," he advised me.

"Father, I started a long time ago. Don't you remember how you and Mama told me to stop reading late at night and to put out the light?" He shook his head in disbelief but said nothing.

He made phone calls to those he thought were lonely. He and I often went to visit his friends who were sick or shut in. We made social calls to everyone we could. Through the Association for the Blind and the newspaper, we found out about a number of classes and activities available to the blind. My father was interested in all of them. We were dazzled by the breadth and variety of classes he decided to take. I took him to almost all of them. I had told my father in his hospital room that day that I would take him wherever he needed or wanted to go when he was able, and I would be his chauffeur and secretary. That day, in that hospital room, I would have promised anything to make his life easier. I was the only member of the family who was not gainfully employed or going to school. I had been thinking about going to graduate school now that my children were teenagers, but when this catastrophe overtook us, I put that plan on hold. I felt that the first year of his "new" life might be the hardest, and he would need all the support he could get.

Every day I left my house about eight o'clock in the morning after Judy and David went to school. As soon as I arrived, my father and I sat down together, went over his schedule, and planned activities for the day. I tried to be home by three-thirty when my teenagers came home.

I was surprised at his choice of activities. Never one for games, he now took up a number of them. He enrolled in a bowling class for the blind.

"Sam, your ball went into the gutter," someone told him the first time he bowled. He was confused by this remark

"I didn't know what he meant," my father said later. "The only gutter I knew was on a roof."

He began horseback riding lessons at a local stable. He had not been on a horse since his European childhood. I remembered the horse that had pulled him off by his shoulder and threw him to the ground. My father still showed us the scar on his shoulder.

"Would you like to take lessons, too?" the stable owner asked me. "I won't charge you."

I looked at the horses. They seemed so big and frightening. I wondered about asking for a pony, but decided against it.

"No thank you," I said. I waited each week while my father mounted his horse and rode away to have his lesson. Those lessons stopped after several months when the stable could no longer supply the extra teachers. More than twenty years later I happened to meet Mary, his riding teacher. She remembered him well.

"I helped him mount the horse and walked beside him," she said. "We gave him Big Red, who had a little spirit. He enjoyed those classes, and seemed fearless."

Harriet drew my father's attention to a notice about karate lessons for the blind. With interest and anticipation he signed up for a series of beginning classes. It was a strenuous and demanding course made up mostly of younger blind people. One day he returned from class with bruises.

"My partner slammed me down to the ground," he explained. He went on to tell of how he had instinctively used the techniques he had learned and had felled his partner, who was at least forty years younger. Luckily, the injuries were not serious. When Dick, the teacher, injured his knee, the karate classes were discontinued, much to my father's regret. He was very proud of his yellow belt.

Another series of classes he enjoyed was swimming for the blind. Although he never did learn to swim properly, he took pleasure in trying. The water had always been a favorite medium of his, which surprised me, because he had rarely been near a pool or a body of water.

His macramé teacher was a complete stranger who had read about him in the paper. She had called and offered to teach him. I was sure he would refuse her offer, but he said, "Let's try it." His fingers were thick and short. Hands that had once cleaned fish and chopped ice now learned to hold delicate strings and fashion them into designs with small carefully made knots. We were surprised at the attractive belts and wall hangings he made. It was her patient and gentle way of teaching that enabled him to learn to make so many macramé gifts for us all. His hands loved to be busy, and although this new craft was so different from anything he had ever done, he found great pleasure in the art of creation. His teacher, Ruth, was a young wife and mother with a family and obligations of her own. She was active in her church, and her children were young, yet she gave time and energy to help my father by sharing and teaching a talent she possessed.

For a number of years the art gallery ran ceramic classes for the blind. Once a week my father went to class to make pottery. He made vases, bowls, and containers in various shapes and sizes. He looked forward to showing us the variety of objects he crafted. Every piece was signed with his first name on the bottom, and each one of us has signed originals. When that class, too, was discontinued, my father was disappointed.

Classes were an important part of his day, but there was still a great deal of free time. Attendance at worship services continued to be an integral part of his schedule. Each morning and evening, he was picked up by fellow worshippers and taken to the synagogue. If there was no one else to take him, one of us in the family would fill in. A number of kindhearted congregants went out of their way to take my father to services. However, after a few years it became more difficult for many of them as they, too, grew older. One day I took him because, at the last minute, his expected ride could not come. As I brought my father to his seat in the shul I overheard one man speak to another in Yiddish, "Sam has four sons-in-law, and none of them will take him to shul regularly."

The speaker of those words was unaware that I knew what he was saying. I was surprised and hurt by that remark. Services were too early much of the year for our husbands to take him. Evening services were at sunset. During late fall and winter the men were still at work. Moreover, none of them were regular worshippers. I had thought that the fellow members of the congregation were glad to bring my father to worship, that it was a mitzvah for each of them, but perhaps it had become too burdensome a task. They were getting older and perhaps needed help themselves.

After a few phone calls among the family, we found that some of our husbands and sons could usually arrange their time to get my father to services and pick him up. Everyone of them wanted to do what he could. Eventually, Dan, my husband, went with him every evening and stayed for services. Esther's son, Paul, assumed a great deal of responsibility as well and found that he enjoyed the prayer service so much that he often went when he did not need to go with my father. All the grandsons filled in when they could.

One time while at prayer service, my father leaned over and whispered to Dan, "My fake eye just fell out. Would you pick it up please?"

Dan, squeamish as he is, dutifully crawled under the seats and searched until he found it. With a tissue he picked up the thin piece of plastic. "Put it back in place," my father requested.

"I can't do that, Dad. It has to be cleaned. Harriet will clean it and put it back for you," Dan answered. We all believed Harriet could do anything. Taking care of his eyes was emotionally hard for her, but Harriet rose to every challenge.

To enliven the days I would frequently invite relatives over for a simple lunch, and we would have "lunch parties." Our guests included Aunt May, who had come to America with my mother when they were both single young women. The two sisters were very different in temperament. We considered Aunt May eccentric. She was also hard of hearing, and her vision was now poor.

"I can see better than she can!" my father, totally blind as he was, said.

My mother-in-law, who liked Aunt May, was often our guest, too. Although serious tensions had existed between my father and the two women earlier in their lives, that was all put aside now. He was naturally gregarious and had a good time teasing, talking, and reminiscing about the past which they had all shared. Aunt May would talk to each of us, but would rarely listen to anyone's response. Actually, all of them were hard of hearing. In the midst of the babble, it seemed that everyone talked, and no one listened. I often felt that I was in the middle of my own Mad Hatter's tea party.

CHAPTER FIVE

European Childhood

I was filled with wonder about my father's ability to pick up the pieces of his shattered life and fashion those shards and bits into a whole new existence. How did he find the spirit to surmount the disaster that had fallen upon him with no warning—to see the world in all its color one minute and to gaze into a void the next? What had enabled him come through a senseless, brutal attack that maimed him so cruelly? From where had come the strength to find again a joy and zest for living? Was it the struggles and dangers of his youth that had prepared him? What was his secret and what could I learn from him? I began by asking him questions.

I knew he had been born in a little village called Naselvitza in Poland in 1900. It must have been a tiny place because I could not locate it on any map. By the age of ten he worked in the family business selling milk, cheese, cream, and butter.

"We went to Klimentov, a market town, every day with our horses and wagon," he explained. "It was maybe an hour away from our village. We sold milk in big metal cans to our customers. We sold to stores and to private people. We had to be back by 11:30 because the cows were milked at noon, and we wanted to watch."

I was puzzled. "Didn't you milk them yourselves?" I asked

"Those weren't our cows," he answered. "They belonged to the landowner. He was rich. He had so much land you couldn't believe it. We bought the milk from him and sold it. We wanted to watch his people milk the cows—nobody should put water in the milk. I remember like today how I watched that they should wash the cows so they would be clean. I walked around the barn and watched them every day. When they were done milking, they poured the milk into big cans. We had a measuring stick to measure how much was in it."

It seemed incredible to me that such a young boy, perhaps twelve or thirteen by then, should have so much responsibility. As he told me of his childhood, there was no self-pity. He was completely matter of fact. He enjoyed describing the world he had lived in. "Every day we took the milk to the city with our wagon and a pair of horses. They were good horses, very good horses. Oh, you don't see horses like that. One horse was so smart and strong. When we got stuck in the mud after a rain, he would bend down his knees and pull the wagon out of the mud, and the other horse, he would pull him out, too. We took good care of our horses. We gave them good food, very good food. We took better care of our horses than some people are taking care of their children. When we got back from the city we took the horses to the pasture so they could walk around and eat. Many times I went in the pasture. I wanted to get up on the horse and sit on him. I patted him on the knee, and he bent down. He knew I was too small to get on him unless he bent down. One time I was sitting on him, and I hit him a little."

"Father, why in the world did you do that?"

"I don't know. You know how young kids are. It was just a little slap, but the horse didn't like that. He turned his neck around, and he took me by the shoulder and pulled me off. I still have he scar on my shoulder where he grabbed me. Then he stood up on his back legs over me. I was laying on the ground, and I thought it was 'Goodbye Charlie.'"

"He could have killed you," I said.

"Oh sure, he could kill me. He had iron shoes on his feet. But he didn't touch me."

I could picture the scene in my mind: my father lying on the ground, the "very good horse" he admired, angry enough to throw him, upset enough to rear up on his hind legs as my father lay before him. But not angry enough to kill him.

"Did you ever try to go up on him again?"

"From that time on, I didn't try to sit on him again. I wasn't taking any chances. A horse is a horse. He still pulled the wagon for me every day, and we got along."

Selling dairy products didn't bring in enough money. The family supplemented its income by buying chickens or eggs from the nearby farmers and selling those, too, in the market at Klimentov. Once they were in the city, they might buy rolls to sell to their neighbors when they returned to their little village.

"In Klimentov, we bought a dozen white rolls from a baker. They would give you three extra rolls if you bought a dozen. We would sell the rolls to the people in our village, but we would keep the three extra rolls. Boy oh boy, those rolls were so tasty. You haven't got no idea." He smacked his lips together in remembrance.

My father's family also had a little grocery store in their kitchen. He said the whole grocery store was worth five dollars, maybe less. They sold flour, sugar, some potatoes, eggs, just a few items. Another means of earning money involved buying a portion of the landlord's harvest. My father, along with his cousin, Paul, and other family members, watched the ripening fruit trees in the orchard. They stayed overnight among the trees to make sure no one stole any fruit. The family put up a little shack for some of the watchers so they could take turns sleeping in its meager shelter.

My father had four brothers and four sisters. The whole family lived in two first-floor rooms in a house that contained several other apartments. Right outside their door was a well from which they filled their barrels with water for drinking and cooking.

He said, "We had trees and land all around us." He lowered his voice. "You know when you have to go to the bathroom, you have to go where there are trees."

I was astounded when he told me that his family did not even have an outhouse, nor was there electricity, none of the amenities we take for granted. When I told him that it seemed like a difficult life for his family, he assured me they were better off than some people. "We had a real floor, not a dirt floor."

Although his family did not have much money, he said they had plenty of good food. "We had a big breakfast every day—cabbage borscht with potatoes. The potatoes were cooked and cut up or mashed with cream. It was delicious. We had sweet cream butter, sour milk so thick you could cut it with a knife. The buttermilk was heavy, like cream. A glass of it in hot weather—mmm, it was delicious."

He relished talking about the food he remembered from his childhood. He licked his lips, and I enjoyed the gusto with which he described the food. He called coffee "kava" or "chicory," and told me how delicious were a cup of steaming kava and a thick slab of his mother's bread covered with sweet butter. Supper might consist of potatoes cooked with milk. His mother made bread every week. If part of it became moldy before the week was out, they would cut off the spoiled part and eat the rest.

Very often, itinerant peddlers stayed with my father's family overnight. They always received a good supper of borscht, potatoes, milk, kava, and bread. Sometimes there were as many as four or five of these traveling salesmen staying overnight. No one charged them money because everyone knew the peddlers barely made a living.

"Where in the world did these peddlers sleep if you only had two rooms and there were nine children in the family?" I asked

"One of the rooms was big. They slept on the floor. It was a real floor, not just dirt like almost everyone else had," he said. "They liked to stay at our house overnight. Everyone wanted to stay with Moshe Naselvitza. That's what they called my father."

My father explained to me that there were many men with the name Moshe. Using the name of the village after his father's first name would more easily distinguish his father from others. Last names did not seem to be used as often.

"We had two horses and a cow of our own," he continued. "We didn't want to always drink the milk from the landlord's cows. We wanted our own milk."

On the Sabbath, services were held in his family's home. The little village was too small to organize and support a synagogue The Torah was kept in a special place in his house. The worshippers came from nearby villages. He said there were often as many as fifteen or twenty people for prayer service. On Saturdays, Moshe led the prayer reading for the morning service. Immediately afterward, everyone was invited to the Kiddush. My grandfather and, Ita, my grandmother, served cakes and schnapps. They did this every week. No one paid them. They were the philanthropists of the village. Ita was the money manager in the family of eleven. She must have been astute and unusually capable at stretching their income. The family and all visitors were well fed, and Sabbath worshippers were treated generously.

I once asked my father if his family was ever mistreated by Gentile neighbors, or if there was violence in his village. He said that sometimes there were reports of pogroms in nearby areas, and fleeing Jews would take shelter with his family. But my father emphasized that his own neighbors were respectful of his father, Moshe Naselvitza, and the family. He spoke with quiet pride. "Our family was known for being good-natured. My father was never angry at people. Our Polish neighbors knew they could borrow a few rubles from my father. He never fooled people. Our neighbors had confidence in us. My father treated people right. My childhood was good, very good."

CHAPTER SIX

Leaving Home

As my father grew into his teens, he assumed more responsibility. He walked through the little village buying chickens, flour, eggs, and sometimes a calf. He could pick up an eight-day-old calf and tell how much it weighed. Often he bought a calf from a neighbor and carried it home. The next day he went to the market in Klimentov to sell it, along with the other commodities he had purchased. Sometimes his family kept the calves they bought and had them slaughtered by a shochet. The skin and the hind quarters were sold. The forequarters were kept for the family to eat because only those parts are kosher.

His responsibilities at home included taking care of his six younger brothers and sisters. He was the third of the nine children. His two older brothers had already left the country several years earlier, leaving him the oldest one still home. His brother, David, was in South America, and Max had gone to the United States.

My father was a big help to his mother. He sang songs to keep the little ones amused. I was surprised because I hadn't known he could sing.

"You never sang to us when we were little, did you?" I asked.

"No," he answered. "I didn't." I should have known that working to support all of us consumed most of his time. He was up well before the rest of us, stoking the coal furnace, so that we children and my mother would be warm when we got up. He chopped ice early in the morning, preparing the fish for the day's customers. It was late when he came up for supper after he closed the store. Sometimes at night he would help my mother scrub clothes on a washboard in the bathtub. No, he didn't have time to sing for us.

My father's family knew of pogroms in the surrounding villages, of violence against Jews in nearby communities, but my father repeated that their neighbors respected them and liked them.

My grandfather had often helped the gentile villagers. They would not, my father claimed, allow harm to come to Moshe and his family. My father said that he and his family felt safe in their village of Naselvitza. They felt no sense of danger, no sense that the violence swirling just beyond their small village could quickly descend upon them. They did not understand that there might come a time when their friendly neighbors could do nothing to protect them.

The unrest and turmoil of the times grew worse. Russia dominated Poland. The Cossacks, a group of daring horsemen and mercenary soldiers who were a law unto themselves, rode through small villages and the countryside terrorizing people. When my father was about fifteen years old, Cossacks riding big horses came thundering through the village. From their doorway, he and his bearded father watched the amazing horsemanship of the Cossacks.

"They were going so fast you could hardly see the horses—maybe fifty miles an hour they were going. One Cossack saw us standing at our door. He stopped his horse so fast the horse stood up on his back legs. One shot, and the Cossack killed my father. Me, he never touched. You couldn't do anything."

I thought about my father witnessing the murder, about his mother, Ita, suddenly widowed, about the fatherless children, about an act of violence without meaning, and I was filled with rage.

"What about a trial? What about bringing that murderer to justice?" I had asked.

He had laughed. "There was no such thing as a trial, especially for Jews. The Cossack said my father was a spy, and that was why he killed him. That was the end of it."

When I heard the story of the Cossack shooting my grandfather, I was struck by the similarity of the words used by my father and his father before him: "My neighbors like me. They wouldn't hurt us. They wouldn't let anything bad happen to us." The words were spoken 47 years apart by Moshe Naselvitza Schafer in Naselvitza, Poland and Sam Schafer in Rochester, New York. Both men demonstrated the same confidence and trust in the people around them.

I pointed that ironic coincidence out to Esther. "They were both wrong, weren't they?" she said.

The following year, 1916, the Russians were conscripting all able-bodied young men into the Russian army. It meant a life sentence of servitude to a government that was hostile to Jews. Once in, getting out of the service was almost impossible. A government official served my father papers to join the army. My father had three months to get ready. He was sixteen years old. Instead of preparing to join the army, he fled and went from village to village, avoiding the police, whose job it was to find "deserters." He asked farmers if he could help them in return for a meal. One time he saw soldiers searching a nearby area. He ran across some fields and hid in a barn, jumping into a haystack and burrowing down as far as he could. As he jumped into the hay, he saw that a pitchfork leaned against the wall, and immediately he realized his hiding place could be dangerous.

From inside the haystack my father could hear the police enter the barn. He heard the pitchfork taken from its place. He held his breath as the pitchfork plunged into the hay. As he lay tense and alert, he tried to decide whether to run if he were discovered or to stay and fight. Again, the pitchfork was thrust into the hay, narrowly missing his face. The third time that the pitchfork plunged into the haystack my father said he could feel the tines touch the skin on his back, but the force of the thrust was already spent. The tines never pierced his skin. Apparently, the police decided to move on and left the barn. My father waited ten minutes to be sure the police were gone and were not tricking him. Then he emerged.

He returned home exhausted, uncertain what to do next. He could not survive running and hiding from village to village My father's mother, Ita, decided what her teenage son must do. She knew that she must send him away. "My mother sold everything she had," my father said. "She had to pay 50,000 marks to smuggle me over the border to Galicia and then to Germany. That was a lot of money. She sent me away. One night she told me, 'Shlomo, it's time for you to go.' I put my head on her shoulder. I didn't open my eyes. I knew how she felt. Her arms were around me. She said, 'Don't ever come back and never write.'"

He told me this seventy years after it had happened, and he began to weep as he described their last embrace and her final words to him. Then I started to cry. We both sat there sobbing, I thought of this remarkable woman whom I had never known or seen, She must have believed a better life is worth untold risk and sacrifice. I said to myself, I am part of this grandmother of mine. I will think of her courage and love. I am glad she and I are forever bound by the ties of blood across time.

My father left in the darkness of night to go to a boarding point. A boat made to carry perhaps twenty people was filled with more than double that number. Other young boys fleeing the country crowded into the small craft which took them to Galicia (Austria). Once safely there, his next step was to take a train to Germany. My father had no money for the train trip, but he boarded the train and lay under the seats. The conductor went through each car collecting tickets.

"I waited until the conductor passed by, and then I came out and sat down with everyone else," he said. "Nobody told the conductor I was under the seats. Maybe they knew I was a deserter, and if I was found out I would be shot."

When he told me the story of his escape from Poland at the age of sixteen, I found it hard believe that he could handle the dangers and uncertainties with such presence of mind. "If you had no money," I asked, "what did you do when you got to Germany?"

"I got off the train in Berlin. I walked around the train station, listening to people talking. I was trying to hear if anybody was talking Yiddish. I heard some people talking Yiddish, and I went up to them and I said, 'I am hungry. I haven't got no money, and I haven't no place where to sleep.' They said to me, 'Go to 55 Viesenstrasse. They will take care of you.' I'll never forget that address. I went there."

My father slept on springs with a blanket for a covering. He said it was fairly comfortable. He could not remember who ran the house, but it must have been a Jewish organization. At 55 Viesenstrasse he met other boys and soon found a small group like himself, religious boys who had left home to escape the army. They were a little older than he, and they knew he had no money. They took him under their wing. The boys went out to eat and always took my father with them and paid for him. He did not want to eat too much, because he was afraid they wouldn't take him along, so he just ate enough to keep alive.

"I was always hungry. For over three years I lived like this," he said.

He and his friends were standing around the railroad station one morning, when they were asked if they wanted to shovel coal into the train. Their payment would be all the coffee they wanted and all the bread they could eat. They began shoveling coal. Afterward when they all sat down to eat, he ate all he wanted for the first time since his arrival in Berlin.

A young disheveled man approached the boys as they sat and ate. He took out a knife and said, "If you don't give me something to eat, one of you will get hurt."

"We told him to sit down with us and eat all he wanted," my father said. "I knew what it was like to be hungry."

When I asked my father what he thought of Berlin he said, "I never saw such a beautiful city. Unter der Linden was the biggest, widest avenue I ever saw. The streets were so clean you could eat off them."

My father acquired a passport with the help of a Zionist organization. He planned to go to Palestine. Right at that time England closed the immigration to Palestine, and he was told they would never open it again. He waited a while, and then he started sending registered letters to two uncles in Utica, New York, and to his brother, Max, in Rochester.

CHAPTER SEVEN

The Consulate

My father's letter-writing campaign brought the hoped-for response. His uncles and his brother sent him 25 dollars and a ticket to America. The next step was to get his visa stamped at the consulate. Impatiently, he awaited word on what day he needed to appear. A year crept by before he received notice to go to the consulate—a year in which he and his friends supported each other's dreams. When the day finally arrived he got up early in the morning.

"I thought I would be first in line because I got up so early," he recalled. "The line was already out the door when I got there. I waited in line all day. When it was my turn next, I went into the consul with the ten dollars it cost for the stamp. I had nine American dollars and one Canadian. The consul wouldn't take it. He said it had to be all American dollars. The two guards shoveled me out of the way and out the door, and it was 'Goodbye, Charlie.'

"I walked back and forth in the hall. I didn't know what to do. I didn't have any more American money. I looked in the mirror on the wall, and I saw my face was all red. I kept walking back and forth. A good-looking young man, maybe thirty years old, was there in the room. He was dressed beautiful in a white suit. He sees me walking back and forth. He asks me in German, 'Vos iss los?' (What is the matter?) I told him nothing was the matter, because I didn't want to bother him with my troubles. He saw I kept walking back and forth. He asked me again, 'What is the matter? Maybe I can help you.' When I heard him say, 'Maybe I can help you,' I stopped walking back and forth, and I stood still. I told him what happened, and I showed him the money. I told him I didn't have another American dollar.

"The man pulls out an American dollar. He wanted to give it to me. I didn't want to take it because I couldn't pay him. He didn't even want the Canadian dollar. 'I can't pay you. I can't take your dollar,' I told him. He insisted that I take the dollar.

"I wanted his name and address so I could send him the dollar. 'I'll see you in America," he said. 'I'll look you up.' I thought it wouldn't be hard for him to find me or for me to find him—you just go out and look around. I didn't know how big was America.

"When I had the dollar, I didn't stand around talking. I walked right back in the consulate's office, past the two guards like I'm supposed to be there. I wasn't going to ask them could I come back in. They might say no. I said to the man sitting behind the table, 'The other consul send me out to get an American dollar,' and I put the money on the table. They didn't know what I was doing there, but the consul saw the money on the table, and he put the stamp on the visa. Don't ask how I felt. You can't buy for all the money in the world that wonderful feeling I had."

My father related this story several times to us and to the grandchildren, and I was always amazed at his good fortune. "Wasn't he lucky that a kind stranger with an American dollar was there at just the right time?" I once asked Maureen and Paul, Esther's children, who were listening with me.

"It seems hard to believe," said Maureen.

"Do you think it could have been an angel?" asked Paul. "He was dressed in white and he was beautiful." Paul was then in high school, a muscular wrestler, an athlete, who went to prayer services often with his grandfather and was more open to a belief in angels than I was.

Before laughing or discounting his idea aloud, I stopped short. What did I know of the infinite mysteries of the world? Who was the handsome stranger in white? Was he a German world traveler who carried American money in his pocket? Did many Germans carry foreign money around? Was he wealthy enough not to care about repayment although times were bad in Germany? Because he spoke German could I assume he was German? How is it he persisted in questioning my father and did not give up after the first rebuff?

"I don't know if he was an angel," I said.

My father was now ready for his voyage. In his pocket he had his ticket to America that his two uncles in Utica and his older brother in Rochester had chipped in to buy. He had his visa stamped. Now he had to wait for his turn to leave. A few months later he was called and told his turn had arrived. He boarded a ship on the Hamburg-American line, and in two weeks he arrived in America. It was January,1921, and he was not yet 21 years old.

His older brother, Max, met him at Ellis Island, or Kesselgarden as my father called this point of entry. My father was somewhat disappointed by his first look at his new country. Berlin had been so clean you could eat off the streets, he had once said. New York looked dingy and shabby. It was littered with papers and was dirty. Max brought him to Rochester, and helped him find a place where he could get room and board in a house owned by people who had known the Schafer family in Poland. Without delay my father wanted to look for work. Max, a tailor, who worked in a clothing factory, tried to find work for his newly arrived brother. He talked to people in the industry.

Max soon found a job for my father working in a tailor shop owned by a Mr. Barnes, who explained the conditions of the job.

"You will work for four weeks without pay, learning the job. After four weeks you'll get paid ten dollars a week." My father agreed and started work immediately in the clothing shop. "I sat down at the sewing machine, and I put my feet down and touched the pedals. It started to go. I jumped away because I was scared. I never saw an electric sewing machine before. I thought there was a devil in it." He used the Yiddish word, "Dybukk."

"Don't be afraid," said his brother, who had accompanied him to his first day at work. "That's how an electric sewing machine goes. There's no devil here."

My father worked hard for four weeks. After the fifth week he looked at his paycheck and saw that it was seven dollars.

"I went to Mr. Barnes and I told him I only had seven dollars—not ten like he promised. He said, 'Greenhorn, in America they keep a few dollars back in the beginning. Next week you'll get ten dollars.' The next week I saw that I had seven dollars again, and I asked him about it. He said, 'Greenhorn, your work was no good. I had to do a lot of it over.' He gave me a solution. He told me to come in at six o'clock in the morning and get the coal stove going and clean up the place. So I agreed. I came in an hour before everybody else and got the stove going. I swept up the shop and made it look nice and clean. When the people came in to work, they were happy. The shop was warm and clean, not cold and dirty like before when they got to work.

"With the ten dollars I made, I paid five for room and board and the other five I could use for myself. One day a boss from another shop, a different one, came in and walked around. He looked at everybody working, and he came over to me. He asked me how much I made, and I told him ten dollars. He asked me if I would come to him to work for eighteen dollars a week. I asked him, 'Are you joking with me?' He told me no. He told me I would work 48 hours, not 80 or 90 hours a week. I said, 'All right, I'll work for you.' He told me not to say anything about it till the end of the week, after I got my paycheck, and then to tell Mr. Barnes that I was leaving to go to a different job. I waited till I got paid, and I said, 'Mr. Barnes, I'm leaving. I have another job.' He asked, 'Greenhorn, where are you going?' A different name from Greenhorn he didn't have for me. I told him the truth, that I was offered eighteen dollars. He said he would pay me 18 if I stayed. I said, 'You told me I'm not worth ten dollars. How are you gonna give me eighteen?' He answered, 'Okay, okay, you'll get eighteen. Stay.' I told him I promised I would take the new job. 'I'm going to go. I won't stay here.'

"So Mr. Barnes said to me, 'Okay, go.' I left and I started my new job. I worked only one week. The shop was a union shop, and the whole shop went out on strike because of me. I told the boss I want to join the union. The union people said no, they couldn't take me. There were lots of Americans that couldn't find jobs. The union didn't take foreigners. I asked the boss what could I do, and he told me there was nothing for me to do, and he could not do anything either. So it was, 'Goodbye job.'

"I couldn't find work for months. I owed my landlady 150 dollars. I had two uncles in Utica, Uncle Joe Schulman and Uncle David Schulman. They wrote to me. They told me to come to Utica. Maybe they could help me. I went to Utica and stayed with my Aunt Lena and Uncle Joe. I found a job with their help in a big clothing factory on Columbia Street that made boys' clothing. It was owned by a German Jew. He had over four hundred workers in his factory."

My father worked for a couple of weeks at a set salary and then he was put on piece work. He said he really went to town when he was put on piece work. He didn't care how many hours he worked. He was ambitious and wanted to get enough money to get on his feet and pay his debts.

"I worked on the noon hour. I took ten or fifteen minutes for lunch. People took an hour for lunch—not me. At five o'clock people went home. The boss asked me, 'Would you like to stay longer? We have a lot of work.'

"I told him, 'Sure, as long as I get paid I'll stay. It didn't take long, and I was making forty or fifty dollars a week.'"

Although Uncle Joe's son, Paul, was several years younger, he and my father became good friends. The cousins, as young boys, had together been watchers in the orchard in Naselvitza, guarding the fruit that they planned to harvest. In Utica they resumed their relationship.

I never knew what kind of work my father did in the factory. Years later Paul told me that my father was a presser who worked steadily in all kinds of weather, pressing clothes even when the pressing room temperature went up to 120 degrees. "Your father was a hard worker," Paul said.

My father kept at his pressing job for over three years and amassed two thousand dollars in savings. He had long since paid his landlady the money he owed her, and now he was ready to look around for a wife. He could furnish a house and assume the responsibilities of a husband. He told me he had been writing to a girl in New York City. Perhaps he had met her on the ship coming over. Maybe she had moved to New York from Rochester. My father didn't tell me how he knew her.

"I was just friends with her. There was nothing specific between us. We just wrote. I went to New York to see her, and I was very much disappointed. I couldn't believe it was the same girl that I remembered. She didn't look good anymore. I lost my whole appetite."

Instead of staying several days to visit her as he had planned, my father left the next day. She wanted to take my father to the train station, but he declined her offer of transportation. That was the end of it, as my father declared. He returned to Utica and began looking around again. He visited Rochester often. The pictures of him taken at that time show him to be a nice-looking young man of pleasing proportions. His eyes were an unusual shade of blue gray, and his hair was light brown. Like many immigrants from Eastern Europe, he was not tall. His papers describe him as five feet four inches. He never felt short because almost all the men he knew were about the same height. The women were shorter.

There were numerous social events for young Jewish immigrants, and he enjoyed the parties and activities. At one such get together of young men and women, an attractive girl caught his eye.

"I saw a girl. I don't know her name," he told Max, "but her brother has a fish market."

CHAPTER EIGHT

Marriage and Store

Perhaps one enchanted evening he saw her across a crowded room. He told me he first met her at a social gathering at the home of a friend of his brother, Max. He was visiting Max in Rochester, as he often did. He liked this girl's looks, he said. Max knew who my father was talking about. The girl was Kate Oratz and, unfortunately for my father, she was already engaged.

"She's going to be married in a couple of weeks," Max told him. "She's already had two showers."

"She's not going to get married in a couple of weeks," my father answered.

I suppose Max smiled or shrugged. A couple of days after this conversation Max put in a call to my father in Utica to tell him the engagement was off, and there was to be no marriage. He didn't know what had happened, but there it was.

"I'm coming in this weekend to take her out," my father replied.

He never did believe in wasting time. He took the train to Rochester and called on her. She went with him to a moving picture show. She apparently spent no time recovering from the broken engagement. Thus began their courtship.

Kate Oratz had come to America with her older unmarried sister, May. They had been brought over by their uncle, Abraham Stolnitz, who had come to America much earlier with his wife and children. The Oratz sisters already had a brother, Isadore, in Rochester. We called him Uncle Yitzrak.

Uncle Abraham Stolnitz was considered a wealthy businessman by his peers. He had had a successful fish market and was retired by the time Kate and May Oratz came over in 1921 from Ostrow Marzowecka. He vouched that Kate and May, his nieces, would not become wards of the state. Kate and May's brother, Isadore Oratz, had taken over Uncle Abraham's business. That business, too, became successful.

When I looked at pictures of the two sisters, Kate and May, as young women, newly arrived in this country, May seemed more striking. Her features were more chiseled, her hair darker, her expression proud, almost haughty. Kate had a softer look and a milder demeanor. Her features were regular, her auburn hair was wavy. They both had deep brown eyes. They were both attractive, but May apparently did not attract any suitors. The custom in Europe was for the older sister to marry before any younger sisters. Uncle Abraham wanted his older niece, May, to marry first. He spoke to my father, and offered him a sum of money if my father would marry May and forget about Kate.

"I'm not getting married with money," my father said. "I'm getting married with a girl." He turned down the offer.

"Do you think May knew you refused to marry her, even with a dowry?" I asked.

"I think she knew. She used to say bad things about me to Kate."

He pursued Kate and took the train into Rochester every weekend for a year to see her. Finally he took her to Utica to meet his Aunt Lena and Uncle Joe. He said that his Aunt Lena was an exceptional woman, and he had a great affection for his Uncle Joe. Kate liked them from the very beginning, and would always hold them in high regard. She and my father became engaged. They were married in Nathanson's Hall in Rochester, June 21, 1925. My father was 25, and my mother admitted to being two years younger. Maybe she was.

When he first told me this story I was in my teens, and I believed my father was prophetic. How could he possibly know that Kate Oratz would break off that first engagement? Back then, in a romantic blur of emotion, I thought that theirs must have been a love that was destined, a romance that would echo through the halls of eternity. Looking back years later, it seemed to me that their marriage was a mystery. He was a risk taker, bold and outgoing, while she was quiet and afraid to take chances. They were opposite in so many ways, but I knew they shared one vision, although I never heard it discussed. They wanted to give their children a life of opportunity and choices that they had never had and would never know.

From the first, their ship of marriage ran into rough weather. They had moved to Utica because of my father's good job, but work slowed down shortly after they settled in their apartment. He had rented a five-room flat above Nozik's Meat Market on Miller Street. My father had bought and paid for brand-new furniture for all five rooms. He said they were happy as newlyweds, but when work became slow he started to worry. Although there was not enough work to keep the workers busy all day, they were not allowed to leave the building. He was impatient because he had to sit idly for most of the day. Wages for everyone dropped, and he could barely make a living. When my father complained to the boss about how he disliked sitting empty-handed for most of the day, the boss said most people were glad to be working at all, and if my father didn't like the way things were, he knew what he could do. My father did not like the way the boss talked to him. He gave notice and left.

My mother was already pregnant with the first of my three sisters, and now my father was out of work. They wrote to my mother's uncle, Uncle Abraham in Rochester, and Uncle Abraham, once again, came to the aid of his niece. He suggested that my father learn the fish business. He offered to teach him and to help set him up in business. My father came to Rochester alone, and together he and Uncle Abraham found a suitable store on Joseph Avenue. Uncle Abraham had another nephew who wanted to learn a business. He offered to teach them together. The idea was that the two pupils would become partners and run a successful business together.

As soon as he had rented the store with an apartment above it, my father sent for my mother. She was nine months pregnant. Coming to Rochester she wondered if she would have her first baby on the train. Several doctors in Rochester refused to accept her as a maternity patient because she was so far along. When she did find one, it was just in time. My big sister, Marcia, was born one week after my mother arrived in Rochester.

Meanwhile, the fish-business classes went on for the two students. My father said that Uncle Abraham was a tough taskmaster. He described a typical class.

"Uncle was rough with us. He kept saying we were both no good. He told me my fingers were too thick. They were so thick that they could hardly bend. 'You'll never be a businessman. You can't even bend your fingers,' he told me. 'How could you be a businessman?' He told us both we were terrible at cleaning fish. He said the other nephew wasn't any better than I was. He didn't see how we could make good. I figured whatever he's telling me, it's for my own good. He was trying to teach us this way, so I kept my mouth shut. The other nephew couldn't take it. He just left, and we didn't know where he went. Much later, I found out he went to New York City to work in a fish market. He did very well. In New York, people get tips and get paid good.

"I was still trying to learn everything about the business when the uncle died. I was alone like a fish out from the water, but I kept on working by myself. I learned while I worked. Kate came downstairs to the fish market and helped me. Then we worked together."

In the midst of this difficult situation, May, the older sister, came to live with them. I never did find out why she made the move to my parents' apartment. When I knew her during my childhood, she was a jealous person always making disparaging remarks about most people, including us.

"She made my life miserable," my father said. "She said I was uneducated and common. She told people that she worked hard to keep our place clean, that she was always trying to help Kate with laundry and cooking. Masha (Marcia, the oldest of us) was a little baby, and to listen to May you would think that she raised her by herself. She told everyone she took care of the baby all the time."

"I don't know how you could handle it, Father," I said. "Aunt May used to jangle my nerves after two minutes in her company. Didn't you say anything to Mother?"

"I didn't want to say anything because I thought Kate would feel bad. I kept my mouth shut."

My Aunt May with her difficult personality, did not find a husband here, and in 1927 she decided to go back to Europe, to her native village.

"She went back to Poland to look for something. She found something," my father said.

From my father's voice I could tell that he thought the "something" was not too good. Aunt May returned from Poland a married woman. Her new husband, David, arrived in Rochester a short time later. Unkind rumors circulated that Aunt May was much older than her new husband. When she was in her eighties, Aunt May told me that no one knew she was about ten years older than Uncle David. It was classified information that actually was public knowledge. One relative surmised that David had wanted to come to America, and marriage to an American citizen was an efficient way of achieving this goal. Aunt May never heard those rumors, or she ignored them. She was very pleased with her status, and she made it clear that her new husband was a very well-educated, pious man, far above all the men in the neighborhood, especially my father.

Uncle David was a shochet and a mohel—he was a ritual slaughterer and he performed circumcisions—two vocations I found disconcerting grouped together. Wielding a knife skillfully was important in both activities. When Uncle's hands got shaky he didn't know enough to retire, and we worried about the outcome for some of his tiny clients. For a long time my parents deferred to Uncle David's opinions in many matters because of his superior religious education. For instance he believed he had a remedy for a wart that grew in the middle of my cheek. He needed the fresh blood of a dove to get rid of it. As a ritual slaughterer he knew how to obtain the bird and its blood. He killed the dove in front of me and then applied the blood to my cheek. My mother tried to calm me during this medical procedure. When the wart remained, Uncle suggested another nostrum. Urine was applied to my cheek. I had no idea from where it came or whose it was. Eventually my mother took me to a dermatologist.

To strangers Uncle David appeared kind and generous. His wife soon found that he was tightfisted and begrudged her spending money. At every opportunity, he pointed out that we girls were not observant enough, and our parents were derelict in their religious duty. When we were a little older we ran in the opposite direction when we saw Uncle, mainly because none of us wanted to be caught in his warm and overly tight embrace. But all that was years later. When he first came to this country Uncle David and my aunt looked to my parents for help.

Despite my father's shortcomings, Aunt May and Uncle David moved in with my mother and father and baby Marcia. They must have been comfortable because no effort was made to find a place of their own. Even when Uncle David found lucrative work, they continued to enjoy the free Schafer hospitality. My father finally felt he had to speak up. "Katie, we're supporting two extra people. He's got a good job. They should start to pay us a little something. It isn't right for them to expect us to support them."

My mother spoke to her sister, and it was shortly after their discussion that my Aunt May and Uncle David found an apartment of their own—not for long, though. In 1930, the year I was born, my father bought a larger store that also housed three apartments. My Aunt May and Uncle David moved into the first floor apartment behind the store. After several miscarriages Aunt May finally carried a son full term. My cousin, Emanuel, was born in 1932. He and I played together until my uncle decided I, and indeed no one, was religious enough or good enough to play with his son.

It was here, at 584 Joseph Avenue, that I grew up.

CHAPTER NINE

Fish Market

We lived above the fish market, and I never even noticed the smell.

My three sisters and I were known as the Schafer girls, and we worked in Schafer's Fish Market from the time we could reach the cash register. Our small apartment over the market faced one of the busiest streets in Rochester. Through the big window by my sofa bed. I could look out over Joseph Avenue and watch the people and horses go by. I could look across the street into the large windows of the Lincoln branch of the public library and observe people as they chose their books. I could hear the clanging of bells as the streetcar stopped at our corner to let people off and to take on new passengers. Sparks flew as the streetcar stopped.

Every night my sister and I pulled out the couch in our living room, the "front room" we called it. The couch turned into our double bed, and sometimes in the middle of the night, I woke up cold because Marcia had the whole blanket. Esther and Harriet, my two other sisters, slept in a real bedroom, and our parents had the other real bedroom.

Living on such a busy street, it was easy to go shopping. We went to Simon's creamery next door for milk, butter, and cheese. At Applebaum's Kosher Meat Market down the street we bought meat of every kind, mostly chuck, sometimes shoulder steak, once in a great while veal chops. My mother bought meat to hand grind into hamburgers. The fruit store a few doors away had fresh fruits and vegetables. We ate whatever was in season. The most exotic fruit was pineapple. Sophisticated ways to ship produce and preserve freshness were years away. Close by were a number of bakeries, and we bought bread, rolls, cakes, pies, and, on Friday, challah (Sabbath bread). Sometimes my mother sent me to buy yeast at Sands' Bakery so she could bake her own cakes and kuchens. She made the best blueberry kuchens in the world. I wish I had asked her for the recipe.

There were almost a dozen fish markets on the avenue. The huge plate glass window of our store had "Schafer's Fish Market" printed in big white letters. We carried a wide assortment of fish. Glittering whitefish came from Lake Erie and Georgian Bay in Canada. There were flounder, round and flat as big dinner plates, silver scaled bass with their mean mouths, and bony trout. My favorite were the mackerel, so beautifully patterned and slim-bodied. There were whiskered catfish, pink-fleshed salmon, and ugly carp. Huge slabs of halibut, pale, wide-eyed yellow pike and blue pike—all lay on beds of chopped ice, in wooden boxes, side by side on a raised platform. As soon as I could write, my father sat down with me and told me what kind of fish and how much to order from Globe Fish Company in Boston or the Atlantic Fish Company and all the other suppliers. Fish was plentiful, healthful—and inexpensive. Haddock was 25 cents a pound and whitefish was about 60 cents a pound.

"Fish is brain food," my father often said to his customers. "If you eat fish every day like me, you'll be smart like me."

At home we always had fish in the icebox. My mother baked whitefish, pickled salmon trout, broiled salmon, fried haddock, cooked smelts or pike, and made sweet-and-sour pickerel. Every Friday she made gefilte fish.

"Ice, Ice," yelled the iceman. He came every other day in a horse-drawn wagon full of big blocks of ice, with indentations showing where they should be cut for differing weights of ice.

The horse knew the route well and stopped at our store automatically. In the store window was a diamond-shaped card with numbers in each corner—25, 50, 100, 150. Those numbers showed the number of pounds of ice needed that day. The iceman's customers all had these cards in their windows and turned the cards so that the amount wanted would be uppermost on the card. The iceman cut the big blocks to the correct size and then, with his huge ice tongs, would swing the block onto his rubber-padded shoulder and bring the block into the store, making several trips if necessary. The children in the neighborhood, including my big sister, Marcia, would clamber onto the back of the wagon when the iceman was in the store. They hastily picked up the slivers and chips of ice that fell to the floor of the wagon when he sawed the ice. They loved to suck and chew the pieces. My father could have arranged to buy the ice already chopped, but that would have cost more money, so he chopped the ice himself and shoveled it into the wooden boxes of fish.

We had a round-faced scale that hung from the ceiling by a thick metal chain. Below the scale and attached to it was a shallow pan into which we slid the fish. The hand on the face of the scale pointed to the number of pounds and ounces the fish weighed, and we figured out the total cost. We didn't know anything about calculators. We didn't even have an adding machine. Most of the time I had to use pencil and paper to figure out the total, but not my father, who could figure out anything in his head.

In the store there was a buzzer in the wall that my father would push when there were more customers than he could handle. Upstairs, when we heard the strident call for help, one or more of us would drop whatever we were doing and rush downstairs. We tripped over each other trying to get there as fast as we could. If he thought we weren't fast enough getting down, he would give us a "look." "Nu, what took so long?" he would say, A glare from him or even a disappointed look would reduce us to a state of dejection.

I had many jobs in the store. My father showed me how to wrap fish for the customers, and he taught me how to make change. Our cash register didn't tell how much change to give. My father never did figure out how to put the tape in the cash register, so it didn't tell us anything. It was just a place to keep money.

When I was a little older I learned how to scale and clean the fish. I would hold the fish by the head, and use a tool to scrape off the scales.

I became so fast at it that fish scales would fly everywhere—my hair, my face, my arms, even my clothes. I then cut off the fins and the tail, slid the knife down its belly, took out the insides, and finally cut the fish into the number of slices the customer wanted. If there were fish eggs or roe, I saved it for the customer because fish eggs were a delicacy. A quick rinse under running water, and the fish was put into a pan ready to be wrapped. First the fish was wrapped in a piece of specially ordered white paper, and then it was wrapped in newspaper that I had laid out on our wrapping table. When we were not busy waiting on customers, I sometimes spent an hour or more spreading newspapers neatly on our wrapping table.

"The customer is always right" was our store's motto, and my father repeated this often. He also explained to us that it was necessary to understand our regular customers and to know what they wanted even before they knew. I watched as he would tell a very particular housewife, "I got some whitefish in the cooler. It came in two hours ago, and I saved it for you," or he might say to a penny-pinching homemaker who was not too particular, "Here's a good bargain. I bought too much haddock, and it's gotta get sold today."

Most customers would examine, smell, and even feel the fish (when my father wasn't looking) before a decision was made. If he caught a customer squeezing a fish he would say, "Pleeze, lady, I don't want you should handle the merchandise. It's not good for them."

One time I remember a woman came in and demanded her money back. "The fish smelled bad and looked old," she reported.

"Where is it? Let me see it," requested my father.

"I can't. We ate it all," she answered.

"If it was so bad how could you eat it? I'll give you the money, but I want you shouldn't come back."

"She must be a customer who isn't always right. Is that why you sent her away, Daddy?" I asked my father after she left.

"She's always giving me trouble, always complaining and squeezing the fish. Let her better go to Cantor's Fish Market."

Thursdays and Fridays were our busiest days. No meat on Fridays for Catholics meant big sales for all kinds of fish. Haddock fillets were especially popular. Jews bought whitefish and pike for making gefilte fish, traditionally served on the Jewish Sabbath—Friday night and Saturday. One Thursday, I waited on a white-haired elderly woman who lived several blocks away. She walked slowly, with a slight limp. She wanted a slice of whitefish, and I carefully cut where she pointed. The piece weighed one pound and three ounces. After a rapid calculation in my head I told her the amount owed.

She counted out her money and left, but about a half hour later she slowly limped back with the package of fish and said, "You overcharged me."

Too embarrassed to say anything, I silently unwrapped the package of fish and reweighed it, this time using a paper and pencil to figure out the cost.

"You're right," I told her as I counted out four pennies.

Sometimes an amateur fisherman would try to sell my father his catch of the day. Most of the time my father said, "No." One time a proud fisherman wanted to sell a big carp that he had caught that very morning. The carp swam silently in a bucket of water. After negotiations my father bought the carp, bucket and all, and put a For Sale sign on it. One of our neighbors, feeling that the freshest fish was the one you purchased live and dispatched yourself, bought it. He thought it would be a generous meal for his wife and five children. The family was delighted with the carp. The children filled the bathtub with water and watched the carp glide and turn so much more easily in its larger quarters. Five pairs of children's eyes followed its every movement. When mealtime drew near, the children begged for mercy on behalf of the carp and raised such a clamor that Mr. Roxin agreed to postpone the execution for one day. He vowed that they would all have carp for dinner the following night. The next day when it came time to take the fish out of the water to prepare it for the evening meal, the children gathered around their father pleading for the carp's life. Five pairs of eyes, tearful and sad, beseeched him not to kill the carp.

"Look how he's looking at us. I think he trusts us," said one.

"He likes us. I can tell," said another.

"I'm not going to eat him. I couldn't," said yet another. The two youngest were mournful and silent.

Mr. Roxin, seeing that there was to be no pleasure in eating this particular carp, put the fish back in the bucket and returned it to our fish market.

CHAPTER TEN

Neighborhood

My father could greet his customers in Russian, Polish, German, Yiddish, or broken English. We were surrounded by immigrants, newly arrived, whose English was halting and heavily accented. The shoppers in our store, the neighbors on the avenue, all the store owners, and everyone who lived in the neighborhood were at least bilingual. They spoke their native tongue and broken English. Those who spoke English well were highly respected.

Like my parents, many of our customers were Jewish and had come from Eastern Europe. They had lived in small villages or shtetls. Like my parents, they had fled from poverty, persecution, and danger. Besides their language, the immigrants had brought with them their religion, their customs, and their hunger for a better life for themselves and for their children. Almost all the immigrant parents we knew, no matter where they came from or what their religion, valued education. My father was unusual for his time because he believed in education for women as well as for men. He wanted his four daughters to be financially independent should they not marry (heaven forbid) or should unexpected disaster befall them.

The neighborhood was a mixture of vastly different cultures and ethnic groups, and the stores and houses that lined the avenue reflected this diversity. Tony, who came from Italy, had a barbershop around the corner on Clifford Avenue. There was a red and white striped pole outside his establishment, which was for men only. Almost all barbers charged twenty-five cents for a haircut, a shave, and a dusting of talcum powder. I remember being sent once or twice to the barbershop with an urgent message for my father. The barber was clad in a white jacket, much like a doctor. He slapped a razor against a thick leather strap. I can still picture how thick, white, and creamy the lather looked as the barber painted my father's face with a short, stubby brush. My father preferred Tony to Leo, the Polish barber, a few doors away. Leo enjoyed a reputation as a ladies' man, and was noted for his many young girlfriends, although he was well into his seventies. Perhaps my father preferred Tony because he was a respectable family man.

Drugstores were considered first-aid stations. When my big sister, Marcia, cut her lip badly on the screen door, my mother held a towel to her lip to soak up the blood. Yelling, "Oy, gevalt," she ran to Keilson's Drugstore with her. If I had something in my eye, or a sliver in my finger I went to Relin's Drugstore next door to us. Tearfully I might show Mr. Relin my finger. He was always reassuring and invariably solved the problem. No one thought of going to the doctor except in a dire emergency, although a doctor lived across the street and had an office in his home. When my father's hand became swollen and infected from an ugly cut, he went straight to the drugstore. If the druggist deemed a situation too serious to handle he would advise his patient to consult a doctor. The druggist charged nothing for his services; the doctor charged at least a dollar or two.

Although we went to the drugstore in times of medical emergencies, more often we stopped there for a treat. Almost all drugstores had soda fountains and sold ice cream novelties. We could buy ice cream cones (three cents for one scoop and five cents for two, with or without chocolate jimmies). We also enjoyed Eskimo Pies, Creamsicles, and orange popsicles. My father liked Dixie cups because he could eat them with the little wooden spoon that came with them. My favorite was the Oo La La—ice cream in the shape of an inverted cone on a stick, covered with a thin coating of chocolate, and its flat top liberally sprinkled with crushed peanuts. I always looked at the stick carefully when I finished my oo la la because some of the sticks had the word "free" printed at the top. That meant my next oo la la would be free. Some drugstores made their own ice cream. Nothing was as refreshing on a hot summer's day as dropping by Keilson's Drugstore for a milkshake or ice cream soda, although frappes, Mexican sundaes, and chocolate phosphates were popular with us, too.

The drugstores sold a variety of foreign-language newspapers. Every day my father bought a *Forward,* a Yiddish language daily newspaper from New York City. A large beautiful St. Bernard dog came to the drugstore regularly for the *Abendpost.* He belonged to two elderly German sisters who lived nearby on Maria Street. The clerk would place the neatly folded paper in the dog's mouth, and with great dignity the dog would turn and leave the store. He then proceeded to his home to deliver the paper to his two mistresses.

Cohen's Kosher Restaurant was a mecca for many people, both Jewish and non-Jewish, who enjoyed the ethnic foods served. My mother and father did not believe in eating in restaurants. "You should better eat at home. Why pay Cohen those prices?" my father would say. However, once a year he would go to Cohen's to buy my sisters and me "specials"—a boxed meal consisting of a thick corned beef sandwich on Jewish rye bread with mustard or mayonnaise. It was cut into quarters and came with a kosher dill pickle and a generous amount of thin, crispy potato chips. All this cost thirty-five cents. A "special" was always our first meal after Passover, a week-long holiday in which we ate no bread and adhered to a strict and limited diet.

Morgan's Barn, a few doors away from our store, was actually a stable for horses employed by the city of Rochester for snow plowing, garbage collecting, and street cleaning. There were water troughs all over the city for horses, and one of these large metal containers full of water stood in front of our store. I enjoyed watching the horses drink at the trough. One time a horse broke out of Morgan's Barn and raced down Joseph Avenue past our store. The horse handlers chased, caught, and brought the frightened animal back to the barn. Next door to Morgan's Barn was a little cottage. One spring morning the woman living in that house awoke to find a horse, his head poking through the open bedroom window, peering at her intently.

Half a block away was Platock's Tailor Shop. Mr. Platock, short and round, usually wearing a tape measure around his neck, could press pants, make alterations, and mend tears. When he went out of business, Lou, a seller of fresh poultry, moved into the shop. Luckily, we lived far enough away from Lou's Chicken Store so that we did not hear the chickens clucking or the roosters crowing. Lou's customers came away with freshly slaughtered poultry. The people who lived next door to Lou were awakened about four in the morning each day by the roosters' crowing. The neighbors complained to Lou.

"There ain't nuthin' I can do. When a rooster's gotta crow, he's gotta crow," said Lou.

The tired and hapless neighbors finally complained to the city authorities. The city officials in charge of such problems said that roosters do not crow at four o'clock in the morning. The problem was not resolved until Lou closed the store and moved away.

The most important place on the avenue to me was the Lincoln branch of the Rochester Public Library directly across the street from our store. The branch had a children's section and an adult section, which children could not enter until they were in junior high school. If we needed to use an encyclopedia or other reference book, we required special permission to go into the adult section, which housed the reference collection. Although library rules stated that children could take out only two books at a time, I could easily race across the street before closing time, return the two books I had finished and take out two others. It did not matter that we had no books at home—I had hundreds of books, only they were all across the street. Books offered a glorious entry into other worlds. I was a frequent user, usually going to the library three or more times a week.

The librarian looked very "American" to me. She was fair, cool, and distant. We patrons were mainly immigrants or children of immigrants, and I felt she disapproved of us. She rarely smiled or helped us find books. Once when I returned two books she looked accusingly at me and said, "You didn't read these books. You just took them out two days ago." I was confused and hurt by this accusation.

"I did read them both. I read one to my little sister, and the other one was for me." I faltered and could say no more.

She quizzed me on the contents of the books. "What are they about?" she asked. I was glad to oblige her by going into great detail describing the stories, thus vindicating myself. I was happy when a new librarian replaced her. The new one was helpful and kind, showing me new books and suggesting titles that she thought I might like. She allowed me to use the adult section although I was not yet in junior high school.

Nearby was a dry goods store which sold aprons, underpants, notions, stockings, umbrellas, garter belts, pajamas, suspenders, babies' clothing, and other sundry items. The proprietor repaired umbrellas and, and was therefore known to us as "the umbrella man." A German sausage shop down the street drew customers from all over town.

Further down Joseph Avenue was a shabby store with hundreds of items stocked on shelves in what appeared to be a haphazard manner. The very pious Orgel family who ran the store could put their fingers on any item with unerring accuracy. On one side of the store were toys, crayons and games. On the opposite side of the store were religious items such as menorahs, mezuzahs, skullcaps, books, and candles. It occurred to me that the store exemplified two of the most important parts of its customers' lives—religion and children.

From across the ocean the immigrants in our neighborhood brought with them their religious practices and customs. Important to everyone's life were the places of worship. I remember three imposing Catholic churches not far from us. Saint Michael's looked like a fortress, an impressive stone structure. I watched nuns in long, flowing black dresses with tight, starched wimples walk in and out of the church. On the hottest days of summer they were all covered up.

"Do they have hair?" I asked various friends. I thought not, but no one was sure. I decided they didn't.

The most beautiful church to me had six tall columns across the wide entry and a high bell tower at one side. Way up at the top of the facade was a panel with the carved and painted figure of a woman holding a baby. She had rays of gold emanating from her head. I liked the name of the church, Our Lady of Perpetual Help. I liked saying it to myself, but I whispered it softly so no one would hear me.

There were numerous synagogues in our neighborhood, some quite small, each with its loyal adherents. My father was a charter member of B'nai Israel, a new Orthodox synagogue with a long wide series of brick steps leading to its front entrance. Thick columns graced this entryway. Its membership included many neighborhood people, and was located within easy walking distance of us, which was very important because my father and other observant Jews would not drive on the Sabbath or religious holidays. He served as an officer of the congregation and participated in the politics of its every day life. Because my father enjoyed the congregants and thrived on taking charge, he eventually became president of the congregation. He attended worship services every day and three times on the Sabbath— Friday night, Saturday morning, and late Saturday afternoon. Ten men, (a minyan) were required at each service to perform the prayers. If the group did not reach the minimum number, someone would rush outside to haul in a passing Jewish male over the age of thirteen. In our neighborhood it was not hard to make up the quorum. Women were not allowed to sit with the men in the synagogue; they sat in the women's section which was the balcony, nor could they be counted in the minyan. My sisters and I often waved to our father as we sat with our mother and peered at all the men below. Only very little girls could sit with their fathers.

During the High Holidays of Rosh Hashanah and Yom Kippur, we children spent more time in the synagogue than we did at any other time. Participating in the prayer service on those holidays was an all day affair. The most exciting moment for me came when the shofar (a curved ram's horn) sounded in a series of shrill compelling blasts. Was it a warning to all of us to mend our ways? Was it to alert everyone of

71

the peril surrounding us? Or was the blast to remind us of our ancient heritage stretching back thousands of years? I made sure I was present for the blowing of the shofar.

At other times I slipped into the hallway to talk to other boys and girls milling in the corridor. Sometimes we children, tired of the long service, roamed outside. The boys chased the girls and teased them by picking up chestnut burrs that fell from the trees lining the street. Opening the burrs they extricated the shiny reddish-brown chestnuts and tied each one in the corner of a handkerchief. Twirling their chestnut weapons and threatening to hit us with them, the boys ran after the girls they liked, trying to frighten them. I kept hoping at least one of the boys would chase me, but hardly anyone ever did. After a while we all went dutifully back inside.

The various holidays came only once a year. The Sabbath came every week, but it was more important than all but Yom Kippur. On Friday afternoons well before sundown, the Jewish-owned stores on Joseph Avenue all closed. My father hastened to get the boxes of fish into the walk-in cooler, take the cash out of the cash register, and lock up. He needed to bathe and dress before going to prayer service.

My mother, who worked side by side with my father in the store, took Friday off to work at home, dusting, cleaning the rooms, and scrubbing the linoleum kitchen floor. She would lay newspapers over the clean floor so that it was clean when the Sabbath began. She cooked all day, too, making chicken soup and noodles. She bought a fresh chicken and plucked the pin feathers, then cut the chicken apart, removing the insides, saving the neck and liver. Sometimes she found an egg inside the chicken, and we were all amazed at this phenomenon. She also prepared gefilte fish, chopping the fish by hand in a big wooden bowl, and adding the other ingredients as she chopped. She formed round fish balls and placed them in a big pot of boiling water. On top of each ball of fish she placed a round carrot slice to make the fish look more attractive. The main course was often a roast with "smashed potatoes." We had challah, the Sabbath bread, and for dessert perhaps a homemade sponge cake. My father liked it with a glass of Swee-Touch-Nee tea and two lumps of sugar.

All four of us children scrambled to help my mother, and then we made ourselves look presentable for the Sabbath meal. We made no other plans for the evening because our attendance was required. Before dinner my mother lit the Sabbath candles, after which my father chanted the traditional prayers. In winter when sundown was early we had our Friday night dinner when my father returned from the synagogue, but in summer we ate before he went. Nothing, absolutely nothing, altered or interfered with the Sabbath rituals. I came to understand later, that the Sabbath was a framework for our lives, one that was to shape and mold our destiny more than I ever would have imagined.

CHAPTER ELEVEN

Christmas Memories

I knew about Christmas from watching *A Christmas Carol* when it played at our neighborhood theater, the Empress. Even before that, I knew it was a cheerful time of year, a happy holiday that brought smiles to people's faces, and friendly greetings to everyone's lips.

When I went downtown with my mother I stared at the decorations in Sibley's, McCurdy's, Formans, Edwards, and all the other stores. Their windows, alive with sparkling lights, and colorful scenes, displayed beautiful mannequins wearing elegant clothes. Inside the stores, garlands of evergreens festooned the walls. Wreaths hung everywhere. Little twinkling Christmas trees graced the counter tops. Beautifully wrapped packages with velvet or satin bows showed shoppers how their gifts might look if they would only buy them right then. I longed to receive such gifts. I knew I would open them slowly to savor the excitement and to save the gorgeous paper and bows. On Sibley's fourth floor we marveled at Toyland—a series of dioramas of holiday fun, storybook figures, and winter scenes.

I didn't tell anyone how much I loved Christmas because I wasn't Christian, and most of the people I knew weren't either. I didn't think I would ever have Christian friends because my parents discouraged it. "If you have a fight with a Christian, she will start to call you names. She might even hurt you," they said. I knew that each of my parents had fled to the United States to escape persecution and danger. My mother told us (when we were much older) how she and her sisters huddled in the cellar of their small home in Poland during pogroms. Marauding villagers ran through the streets looking for Jewish girls to rape. My father told us he had witnessed the murder of his father from the bullet of a Cossack. As a child I only knew that my parents mistrusted Christians. I saw that they were respectful and courteous to all our customers, and my father joked and laughed with everyone. Still, they warned us that harm might befall us if we tried to make friends with other kinds of people. It seemed best to say very little of how much I liked Christmas.

During the holiday season I enjoyed listening to Christmas carols on our radio, a floor-model Philco. The carols all had such lovely melodies. My favorite was "Little Town of Bethlehem." It filled me with a sense of mystery and wonder. Another favorite was "Oh, Holy Night," the way Kate Smith sang it on her radio show. Sadly, it was the carols that caused my friends and me big worries every year. During the month of December all we sang in music class at Number Nine School were Christmas carols. Should we Jewish children sing the carols, too? Would lightning strike us if we did? If we didn't sing would our music teacher grow angry? Would we draw attention to ourselves? Would any of our classmates pick fights with us on our way home if we didn't sing? I asked some of my Jewish classmates what they were going to do.

"I'm not going to sing any carols, but I'm going to make believe I'm singing. I'll move my lips, and no one will know the difference," Irwin answered. He demonstrated by forming words with his mouth silently.

"That's a good idea," I said. "What are you going to do?" I asked another.

"I'm going to sing everything except the parts we shouldn't sing," Estelle said. "I'll sing 'Away in the manger no crib for a bed, the,' and then I'll keep quiet until we come to 'sweet head'."

"That's a good idea," I said. Somehow or other we got through music class.

When I was a child, Christmas represented for me a great big party that everyone else was invited to, and I was on the outside looking in—except for one year. Maybe my sister and I had heard the poem, "The Night Before Christmas." Maybe we had heard a radio program during December that gave us the idea. Whatever the impetus, we both approached our parents the night before Christmas and begged them to let us hang up our stockings. Marcia might have said that practically every child in the world hung up stockings, and we felt bad that we didn't. Maybe I promised that we would never ask again if we could do it once. Perhaps our mother and father looked at our imploring faces. With unbelieving ears I heard my father say, "All right."

We had no fireplace, mantel, or hearth in our flat above the fish market, but we did have a great big coal stove with an oven on top. Across one side of the top was a metal bar. On this bar Marcia and I carefully hung our thick woolen knee socks.

We slept badly that night. Early in the morning we jumped out of the bed we shared and ran to the kitchen to examine our stockings. They were bulging. Shouting and laughing we took our stockings from the stove and turned them upside down. Out rolled some bright, round oranges, a handful of walnuts in the shell, and some hard candy wrapped in cellophane. We jumped up and down with excitement. We hugged each other in our delight. In my mind's eye, I still see those two little girls jumping with joy. In my ears, I still hear their laughter.

CHAPTER TWELVE

Smoking

My father smoked three packs of Camels a day. Perhaps he started in Europe as a teenager when he and his friends wandered around Berlin. I remember that he always had a cigarette in his hand—even his fingers were stained brown. Only on the Jewish holidays and the Sabbath did he stop because smoking was forbidden at those times to Orthodox Jews. He must have been about 40 when he began having trouble with his legs. They hurt when he walked, and on the Sabbath he walked to shul because driving was also forbidden. He could drive himself anywhere, but not on Saturday. He walked slower and slower.

My father went to the doctor who, after an examination, said, "It's your circulation. Quit smoking."

Ignoring the doctor's advice, my father continued smoking. Walking became so difficult that once he had to stop on his way to shul and stand still, unable to go on. He was closer to home than the synagogue so he managed to get home. He returned to the doctor.

"Did you quit smoking?" the doctor asked when my father finished his complaint.

"No," my father answered.

"If you're not going to listen to me, Sam, don't come here. Save your two dollars for this office visit, and don't bother me."

This time my father took the doctor's words seriously. He wanted to walk again without pain and effort.

"I'm quitting," he said to the doctor, "right now." He left the doctor's office determined to regain his walking legs. It couldn't have been easy after all those years of heavy smoking. He told me how he did it.

He carried a full pack of Camels in his breast pocket. When he felt an overwhelming urge to smoke, he took the pack out of his pocket and held it before his eyes. He demonstrated how he carefully held the pack in his hand and looked hard at it. "Who is stronger—you or me?" he asked the pack. Powerful waves of an intense desire to smoke pounded against him. He ignored them, and spoke to the pack as a warrior to an adversary, "I am stronger." He put the pack back in his pocket without taking a cigarette. Eventually he broke the habit. His health problems cleared up.

Harriet, the youngest of us, doesn't even remember that he smoked. All she remembers are his numerous tirades against the evils of smoking—a habit he forbade his daughters to begin.

CHAPTER THIRTEEN

Groceries

On Saturday nights after sundown the Sabbath ended, and we reopened the store for business, as did most of the other Jewish shop owners. Although the avenue was quiet all day, Saturday, night it burst into life. People thronged the streets, and often a line formed to get in before we opened. Some customers shopped for lox or herring for Sunday breakfast. Others looked for dill pickles or our big black olives from the barrel. We had schmaltz herring and pickling herring in barrels, too. Every day and Saturday night my father rolled out the huge barrels from our cooler to the sidewalk, and lined them up alongside our storefront. Sunday was a busy day, too. Even years later when the neighborhood changed, women came with their husbands or grown sons who drove them to the store. My father enjoyed talking to everyone. He was an excellent salesman, and would frequently point out special bargains "for this week only."

In the late thirties, a trusted salesperson from a large wholesale house urged my father to begin selling groceries in addition to the fish.

"Sam, people are going to want to do more shopping in one store. You have the room here to build shelves and stock items like cereal, bulk food, and canned goods."

"Do you think people will want to buy groceries from a fish market? Maybe they will be afraid that everything will smell like fish," my father said doubtfully

"No, Sam, I don't think anyone will worry about that. Canned goods won't pick up smells, and you always wrap the fish up with plenty of paper, anyway. When you give people their order, put the fish in a separate bag. People will welcome the convenience of buying grocery items when they shop here." The salesman was astute, and my father agreed with him. He recognized a good idea when he heard one.

It did not take long for the carpenters to arrive and cut the wooden shelves right there in the store. We made extra bargains and cut prices during the renovations, in order to help customers ignore the flying sawdust and the noise of the saws. The carpenters measured the wall and nailed the shelves into the wall as high as they could go. My father was barely five feet four inches, and I was catching up to him. He bought a long-handled "grabber" to reach cans on the top shelf. It wasn't easy to grab a can on the top and clench the handles so that the can was firmly held. Sometimes my grasp was so poor that the can came hurtling down on me. I became adroit at ducking Libby's purple plums or Lily of the Valley baby peas as they fell.

We began the grocery line modestly with displays of Maxwell House Coffee, Del Monte peas, and a basic inventory of groceries sent in by the wholesaler. The salesman made up the list of merchandise because my father knew little about what to buy.

We all had new tasks: stocking shelves and making displays in the windows and on all the available floor space. We built pyramids of cans—a pyramid of Del Monte's sliced peaches, another of Campbell's cream of mushroom soup, a large display of Postum, another of Bosco Chocolate Syrup. I varied the height of the pyramids by putting some of the displays on top of a carton. We made price tags out of little pieces of paper and taped these scraps of paper on the top can of each pyramid. I and one of my sisters wrote out the signs because our handwriting was more legible than my father's. I usually wrote as dramatically as I could, putting SPECIAL! TODAY ONLY! on the top can with one or two exclamation points. There the sign stayed until it became too flyspecked or fell off.

Some items such as sweet pickles came in glass jars. Those always went on the bottom shelves. None of us wanted to take the chance of dropping a jar as we lifted it with the "grabber." We had enough to do without mopping up pickle juice and shards of glass. Large cardboard containers of powdered laundry soap like Oxydol or Rinso were also too heavy for high shelves. Kellogg's corn flakes and Wheaties were light enough for any of us to grab from the top. I gave much thought to the placement of our groceries.

My father kept adding new items all the time. He bought fifty-pound burlap bags of dried navy beans, rice, green split peas, yellow split peas, and lima beans. All of these had to be scooped out of the big bags and weighed into one and two pound paper bags and labeled. Spices came in five- or ten-pound containers, and using a little scooper we weighed the various spices into four-ounce packages. It was tiresome, and I was often bored, measuring five pounds of paprika into little paper bags and making sure each bag contained four ounces.

At first none of us could remember all the goods that we had so recently purchased. A customer came in one day shortly after we were newly stocked and asked for spaghetti. I looked at the shelves, and noticed my father was looking somewhat blankly at the shelves. I had the feeling he didn't know what spaghetti looked like.

"We don't carry spaghetti," he said.

After the customer left I kept looking, and I soon spied boxes of Mueller's thin spaghetti on a lower shelf. We should have put it on a higher shelf, I thought to myself. My father was very upset that he had sent the customer away, and he immediately began looking at the shelves carefully, scrutinizing the merchandise. He spent extra time walking up and down in front of the shelves trying to memorize what he saw. He didn't make a mistake like that again.

We began selling soda water. We called it pop. Par-T-Pak was popular. Nehi beverages sold well. We carried Miller's pop, made and bottled in town not too far from our store. In addition to moving big boxes of fish and huge barrels of herring, my father now carried heavy crates of pop to and from our storage room, leaving some in the store for display.

With the expanded lines of products that we sold came more work for everyone. Now we had more cartons to unpack, more incoming orders to check, more bills to pay, more inventory to keep track of, more letters to write about items damaged in shipment or orders not accurately filled. My father worked sixteen or seventeen hours a day, my mother at his side; the rest of us scurrying about at his direction. He enjoyed the added pressures and decided to buy as much as his credit would allow.

"Volume," he said. "We make money on turnover. We can buy cheaper if we buy a lot."

Our back storage room was soon so full of boxes, I could hardly get in to retrieve merchandise for our displays. Still my father was determined to improve our sales. He began visiting the new Star supermarkets, a larger grocery with weekly specials to entice the shopper. There were no Stars in our neighborhood. My father drove to various areas to spot the Supermarket specials and to assess the new competition. He bought as many cartons of featured items at Star supermarkets as they would allow, and as he could pile into his car. Our store became crowded with cartons of the Star Supermarket specials, which he then sold for a penny or two more.

His philosophy seemed to succeed. He watched his profits climb, but my mother was not happy. She did not approve of buying in volume, of spending so much time working. Her own health had deteriorated, and she wanted more time with my father at home. They had both worked with all their strength, but now that she had to slow down, she resented the enormous investment in time and energy my father still expended. As we grew older she began to argue with him openly. I heard her angry remarks and his replies.

"I can't slow down," he said, "The girls need to go to college some day." His answers did not appease her.

"Talking to him is like talking to a wall," she said. She called him stubborn (farakshund). Her anger piled up like storm clouds. Soon she would burst into a flood of invective. He was not deterred, although he was chastened when she turned on him with her shrill words and hostility.

Who's right? I wondered. I believed in the way my father ran his business. I learned from him the importance of constantly searching for

82

ways to improve. My sisters and I learned from them both the value of giving ourselves completely to the task at hand, and we inherited their endless capacity for work. I appreciated my mother's desire for the family to spend time together away from the fish market.

It took years before I came to understand that she had talents and aptitudes that she never expressed. She was lonely when her children began to need her less. She wanted my father to stop working so many hours, to stop buying so much, and to spend more time with her. She needed someone to talk to. We four girls were busy with school, and we still helped in the store. Why didn't I ask her about her struggles as a working mother, her sacrifices, about her hopes? We never talked about feelings or emotions. Could any of us even recognize our feelings?

During my childhood there was never enough time to talk to either of my parents. They were both too involved with the fish business, raising a family of four children, and following the dictates of their religion. As we grew older we were busy with high school friends. Even when I went to the University of Rochester and lived at home, I helped in the store. There was no time to sit down to talk to my mother. She continued to argue with my father. The conflict between them was never resolved.

CHAPTER FOURTEEN

Innocence

After the New York World's Fair of 1939-40, rumors abounded on Joseph Avenue of the wondrous advances in technology that would soon change our lives.

"You can have a movie show in your own house all the time," said Muriel, my girlfriend, as we walked home from school. We were both in fourth grade. "My big brother went to the World's Fair, and he told me all about it. I'd love to see movies every day, wouldn't you? We wouldn't have to go to the Empress."

"We couldn't have movies in our flat," I answered. "Where would we put the guy that runs the projector? There's no place for him to sleep. We don't even have room to set up the projector and a screen. Our flat isn't big enough to have movies going on day and night. Anyway, my mother would never let a strange man stay in our house. I like going to the Empress, so I don't care."

Not wanting to put a damper on Muriel's enthusiasm, I added," Maybe I'll come to your house sometimes to see your show."

"You won't need a projector or anyone to show the movies," Muriel, the movie expert, laughed. "It's going to come out of a box. You just watch the box."

I smiled at Muriel as one would to a foolish and gullible child. "Muriel, your brother is fooling you. It's impossible to see movies in a box." I dismissed the whole idea as a figment of a feverish imagination belonging to Irving, Muriel's oldest brother. He had always been a big tease. It was perhaps five years later that I actually saw a television set.

My lack of worldliness and that of my sisters was evident in every aspect of our lives—perhaps most of all in the area of love, lust, and what we then called the "birds and the bees." I knew nothing about the human body except my own, which I felt was probably not normal. I did have some basic information from my parents, and I imparted this knowledge to Muriel.

"I know the stork brings babies," I said to Muriel as we walked home from school. We were now in fifth grade. "My parents told me all about it when my baby sister, Harriet, was born. The stork drops them off at the hospital, and the mothers go to the hospital to pick them up. The mothers stay there awhile to take care of the new baby before they both come home."

"I don't think storks have anything to do with the baby business. Did you ever see a stork flying around Joseph Avenue or any other part of the city?" I never had, but that did not shake my certainty. My parents told me, so it must be true. We argued all the way to the store.

"I'm going to ask my father right now," I told Muriel. "You can come in with me. Then you'll believe me."

"No thanks. I'll wait outside. I don't like the smell in your store," said Muriel.

My father was cleaning fish when I ran in. There were no customers in the store, and I was glad to have his full attention.

"Don't babies come from the stork?" I asked without preamble.

He stopped cleaning fish for an instant. His face turned a brick red, and he said nothing. I waited, and then I repeated my question. I looked back at Muriel outside, waiting patiently for me to come up with a definitive answer. My father began to mumble something and stopped. He said nothing. This was unexpected and puzzling. I was confused about what to do. He didn't look at me. I waited a few more moments before I realized he was not going to answer me. I walked out of the store.

"What did your father say?" asked Muriel.

"He didn't say anything," I answered. "I think he has a lot on his mind today. I'll ask him another day." I never did.

Perhaps I knew he could not answer. There was so much I did not know, but I sensed that the answers I wanted, my parents could not give. They had been through hardships and danger. Separately, they had left the land of their birth, the love and closeness of a large family, and everything familiar. Out of need, they had adjusted themselves to their changed circumstances with its different customs and its foreign language. They learned English as best they could, twisting their tongues around unfamiliar sounds, unknown words. They would never be completely at ease with the English language, although, in time, they both learned to communicate well even with their heavy accents.

They had faced the new world, and together they had built a life, wresting opportunity from whatever befell them. Their lives had been full of drama and excitement. Maybe I knew all that as a child. Still, I felt they were innocent about what I wanted to know. There was something in the structure of this country that was unknown to them, its attitudes, mores, and openness that I would have to find out about by myself. They came from a circumscribed world, and in my mind they did not know about the wide world beyond. I turned to my two favorite pastimes—books and movies. It was there I might find what I was looking for, there in the magic between the covers of a book and on the screen of the neighborhood theater I might find answers.

CHAPTER FIFTEEN

Movies

Saturday was a day of complete rest at our house. Our parents worked arduously all week, and appreciated the Sabbath. Because they were observant, they followed all the laws concerning the Sabbath, and we learned how to follow them as well. We had a "Shabbos goy" who turned our lights and the stove on and off, and handled other tasks that an observant Jew would not do. Religious Jews would not go to the movies on the Sabbath. Yet there came a time when Marcia and I clamored to go to the neighborhood movies on Saturday afternoons. Why did they allow us to go? We did not ponder such questions for long. With their permission we raced out of door and down Clifford Avenue to the Empress Theater, where we were transported into a magical world of romance and adventure. The movies introduced us to "real" American life. Avidly, we watched the screen to observe how Americans talked, dressed, and behaved in various situations.

We saw whatever was playing. Neither one of our parents went to the movies, and it never occurred to them to screen what we saw. They probably felt that nothing objectionable would be shown in a movie theater in America. Actually they were right. At that time, the Hays Office, a censoring body, made sure that there were no profanity and no explicit sex in movies. There was little, if any, violence. Yet I and the entire audience experienced intense excitement, suspense, and emotion.

We saw America through the lens of the movie camera. There was Gene Autry and Roy Rogers, each singing with their cowboy friends, as they rode through the West. That was how we found out what the West looked like, as our heroes were busily righting the wrongs they invariably found. They and their friends were loyal to each other, to their country, and they spoke out bravely when they encountered villains. And they sang together. We saw the small towns, the big cities, the mountains, the farms, and we never tired.

We first visited the South Seas and other tropical lands with Dorothy Lamour, sometimes witnessing a hurricane first hand. Tarzan introduced us to the jungle. He and Jane lived in harmony with the wild animals, except when a lion or tiger or alligator tried to harm Jane. Then Tarzan engaged in hand-to-hand combat with the beast, and he always came out victorious, although his only weapon was a small knife.

The Empress Theater introduced us to ancient history. My sister and I saw *The Mummy's Hand,* and we screamed along with everyone in the theater when the mummy climbed out of his sarcophagus after thousands of years of entombment and sought vengeance.

"Watch out!" I screamed to the hero, Dick Foran, as he worked underground in the crypt, unaware that the enraged mummy stood behind him and was slowly drawing nearer with arms upraised and outstretched.

"Turn around, turn around," yelled the boy in front of me to our unsuspecting hero as the mummy came closer. Our warnings could not have helped, yet our hero came out unscathed from every unfortunate encounter with the mummy, even rescuing his beautiful lady friend who was also part of this archeological dig.

The brave and the good in every movie almost always escaped permanent harm or injury. Only a priest, a loyal retainer, or a goodhearted underling died trying to help the hero, but that did not happen often. When it did, I was sad, but philosophical because the hero was young, good looking, American, and he had a sweetheart who needed him. During World War II it was different. Then it was noble for the young and handsome to die.

Sometimes movies puzzled us. I held a Kleenex to my mouth to stifle sobs as Vivian Leigh threw herself from a bridge rather than face Robert Taylor upon his return from the war in *Waterloo Bridge.* Why had she done that? Why couldn't she face her sweetheart? In his absence she had been poor and lonely, and had walked along the streets, smiling at men as they passed by. Often her smiles had been rewarded by overtures of friendship, and she and her new acquaintance walked off together. Doubtless, these friendships helped her while away the time. She had believed that her own true love had been killed in the war, so why wasn't she overjoyed to see him when she found he was alive? I could not understand, nor could Marcia, who was four years older. If we both couldn't understand something, we shrugged off our puzzlement and let it go. We did not ask our parents to explain.

Our excursions to movie land lasted at least four hours. There was a main feature, a "B" movie (with lesser known actors), a serial, Looney Tunes or some Mickey Mouse cartoons, some shorts such as Our Gang or Laurel and Hardy, the coming attractions, and the RKO Pathe News or the Movietone News. We could hear the news through the radio, and read it in the newspaper, but we actually could see the news at the movie theater. At the Empress we first saw Hitler inspect his troops and address throngs of cheering crowds. We watched the Hindenberg explode. My sister and I witnessed King Edward VIII's abdication speech, as Wallis Simpson, the twice-divorced American commoner who was the cause of it all, smiled at her royal sweetheart. She was awfully old and not nearly as pretty as Hedy Lamarr. We wondered why he would give up a throne for her, of all people. How could anyone give up being king? My mother thought Mrs. Simpson was a meezkeit (very homely).

Only once, while I was in Marcia's care, did we see a movie that frightened us both too much. In the movie, large crowds of people were angry, disheveled, and yelling about something. I did not like their looks and their shouting. I slid under my seat and sat on the floor.

I pulled at Marcia's skirt and asked, "Is the bad part over yet?"

When she said, "Yes," I sat back in my seat and watched again, only to find that the crowds of angry people were soon back yelling and screaming more loudly than before. Down I went under the seat again.

Finally she said, "I think the bad parts are really over now."

I climbed up on the seat and watched the movie once more. Too late we realized a terribly bad part was upon us. I watched in horror as a coach drawn by four running horses raced through a crowded street of poor unkempt people who tried desperately to get out of the way. A little child could not reach safety fast enough, and I covered my face as the thundering horses galloped over him. The heartbroken mother ran to her child and kneeled beside him. She gathered his lifeless little body in her arms and wept inconsolably. The coach stopped, a nobleman stepped out and threw the mother some coins.

"Is this enough for your wretched boy?" the richly dressed nobleman asked.

I slid down to the floor, and Marcia got tired of my pulling at her skirt. She took me by the hand and we went home. "I didn't like that movie either," she said.

Our mother, surprised to see us so early, asked what was the matter.

"It wasn't a very good movie," Marcia answered and I echoed her.

We never did see the end of *A Tale of Two Cities.*

As a teenager I watched the movies to see when and how young people held hands, and when and how they kissed. I needed to know how to respond appropriately if I were ever in a romantic situation. I noticed that love and marriage went hand in hand, and sweet and virtuous women always reaped rewards. They found love and good fortune. I wanted to find love and good fortune some day.

When I was about 14, I was entranced by a scene in a movie with vivacious June Allyson dancing with Van Johnson or maybe Peter Lawford. They were in a college gym festooned with streamers, balloons, and decorations in celebration of the spring ball. As her dancing partner swept her chastely around the dance floor, she, blonde and sparkling, looked up at him and laughed merrily. They had no cares or duties. I envied her popularity, her ease and confidence, and wanted desperately to belong to such a life and to leave behind the life of the fish market.

CHAPTER SIXTEEN

Library

It seemed that I always knew how to read. From the front window of our apartment above the fish market, I could look across the street right through the plate glass windows of my favorite place on the avenue— the Lincoln branch of the Rochester Public Library at the corner of Joseph Avenue and Clifford. I watched people choosing books from my perch on the window sill.

When I was young I went through the picture books section, with easy words in large print. My parents could not read English well enough to read to me, but that didn't matter. I enjoyed holding the books myself, turning and feeling the pages, some so smooth and others a little rougher to the touch. Most pictures were in black and white, although some books had a frontispiece in color. I liked the *Flicka, Ricka, and Dicka* series and the *Snip, Snap, and Snur* series, with bright red illustrations. I began reading fairy tales and went through all the Andrew Lang tales. I read every version of Aesop's Fables, and the folk tales of every country, and I became acquainted with the mythology and folklore of a great part of the world. Through my reading I became familiar with the allusions I heard others use. I knew about the Midas touch, was determined never to cry wolf, and hoped to meet a Prince Charming.

I devoured animal stories of all kinds—*Black Beauty*, all the Lassie and Silver Chief stories, and the *Jungle Books*. I loved *Dr. Doolittle* and wished I could converse with animals in their own language as he did. We had no pets. Indeed, I was afraid of dogs and cats. My father told me a dog had attacked me when I was a little girl playing in front of the store. He ran out when he heard my cries, and hit the dog with a stick, frightening him away. Apparently a neighbor called the police and reported that my father was abusing a dog. When the policeman confronted my father and asked why he had hit the dog, my father answered, "What would you do if a dog was attacking your little girl?" The policeman and my father came to an understanding, and no one suffered permanent harm, but I was never comfortable around dogs.

As I grew older I began to enjoy adventure stories, making no distinction between boys' or girls' books. *Call it Courage* was a favorite and all of Pease's books, *Wind in the Rigging, Hurricane Weather, Jungle River*. The main characters were resourceful boys, and although the heroes were not much older than I, they were not afraid to undertake challenges, or to venture into territory that was uncertain. Such young people had high moral standards as well. As far removed as I was from the settings of the stories I read, I absorbed their messages.

Stories about America's past beckoned me. A friendly librarian recommended a recent series. "You're going to like Laura Ingalls Wilder," she said. Once I read *Little House in the Big Woods* I could hardly wait for each successive volume. From books such as those, I learned more of this country's pioneer history. Independence and an emphasis on individual achievement were attributes I began to value. I went through all the Louisa May Alcott books, comparing the little women with my sisters and me. I was Jo.

I discovered Nancy Drew and wanted to be like her, blue-eyed and blonde, fearless and adventurous. She apparently could go anywhere she pleased without her father's curfew and restraints. I began to chafe, as did my sisters, at our restrictions.

At twelve or thirteen romances piqued my interest. Singularly innocent by any standards, I looked to books, as well as movies, for clues to boy-girl relationships. The Isabel Carleton series influenced my behavior all through high school and beyond. Isabel showed me that a good and virtuous young woman would repel improper advances, and that men would then respect a girl with high standards and love her all the more. This definitely reinforced what my mother had been telling me all along.

I discovered poetry. I recited strange and wonderful words to myself to hear their sound and rhythm or to see in my mind the image evoked by the language. I recited Sara Teasdale and Edna St. Vincent Millay often. The English language excited me. Almost all the dialogue or narrative, whether written or spoken in movies or books that I heard or saw was standard American. My impressionable mind absorbed the ideas and the words. So pervasive was the influence of the books and movies that eventually I winced when I heard grammatical errors. I imbibed the structure of the English language, and discovered the power of words.

No matter what kind of books I read, I was learning concepts new to me—about this country and other places, about people and what they thought was important. I believed that Good always triumphed over Evil, a belief that stayed with me many years.

I did not then appreciate how hard it was for my parents to struggle with the collision of their culture with America's. The freedom and openness of this country were unknown to them. They believed in its greatness. It had saved them, and they embraced American ideals, but they wanted to keep their values and beliefs, too. I never asked them about the difficulties they must have faced trying to reconcile the differences of the old and the new. I had enough trouble handling my own divided loyalties.

There was a time when I was in my teens that I was embarrassed by my parents' foreign accent, by the fish market and the neighborhood of my childhood. It was years before I understood the meaning of my parents' strength; the vitality and passion of their world and the world I grew up in. It was even more years before I understood how the strands of that world were woven into a rich tapestry that became the very fabric of my life.

CHAPTER SEVENTEEN

Superstition and Minyan on the Moon

"Should I leave more money to the daughter closest to me, or to all my children should I leave the same?"

My father listened carefully to the customer who posed the question, a widow who needed to talk over her situation. He had a friendly way of engaging people in conversation, and customers who came into the fish market would often stay a little while to joke and laugh. Sometimes a customer asked him his opinion on a perplexing problem. My father relished all discussions and social interaction, whether it involved lighthearted banter or serious questions. He often told us, when he got home, about the problems people had and how he helped them.

It was a rare person in our neighborhood who consulted a lawyer or a psychologist. They cost too much. They were hard to talk to. They probably could not be trusted with personal family problems. It was easier to talk things over with a "maven," someone who was known to be knowledgeable about a given topic. It was even better if the "maven" was a "lantsman" (a person who came from the same area). My father was happy to offer free advice. Lack of a degree in psychology, law, or any other field of knowledge would not stop him.

"What did you tell that lady about leaving her money?" I asked when he told us about it.

"I told her that she should divide the money evenly if she wants the children to get along after she dies. If she leaves somebody out or gives one of the children a lot more than the others, there will be jealousy and fighting. If she wants they should be good with each other, give them each the same."

That sounded logical to me. I knew I would feel awful if my sisters got more of an inheritance than I did. Just thinking about it upset me. I would expect them to share whatever they got so I wouldn't be left out. Maybe they wouldn't feel like it, and that could develop into a big battle. Undoubtedly my father was right.

My father was also a source of information on who to call for fixing and repairing anything. If asked, he could recommend an electrician, a plumber, an auto mechanic, a roofer, a mason, even a plasterer. Invariably he could come up with the name of someone for any task.

"Mr. Schafer," a customer might say, "I need a good 'paintner;' he should do my kitchen—nothing else—just the kitchen."

"I know a good 'paintner,' and he won't charge an arm and a leg," my father probably answered.

One recommendation that did not work out well was that of an auto mechanic, Mr. Finkel. He was known to us as Yunomee because he ended all his conversations with the phrase, "You know me."

A troubled car owner might ask Yunomee, "Can you fix me mine car it shouldn't stall?"

"Of course; I can fix anything. How could you ask? You know me."

"Is it going to cost a lot?"

"I never charge enough. That's my trouble. You know me."

"Will you finish the work when you say?"

"When I promise you your car will be done on a Wednesday, it'll be done. Finished. You know me."

Unfortunately, too many of Mr. Finkel's customer's, including my father, found to their chagrin, that he knew too little about fixing cars, and he charged too much for what he knew. Such difficulties did not deter customers from seeking advice, nor my father from sharing information.

The problem was that my father gave me and my sisters too much advice. As we grew older we wanted less of it and more freedom. He still had "Old World" ideas about too many areas of life—religion, family obligations, going out with boys, even going out with girls— and he continued to dictate to us.

I was caught between two worlds. I felt like a person divided into two parts that were constantly at odds with each other. I wanted to be like a "real American," free of all the religious taboos, the dietary strictures, the protective constraints, yet I was always pulled toward my parents' way of living. I wanted to be loyal to their values, too. It wasn't easy, this living with the Old and the New. Even in little ways, the Old World kept cropping up. For instance, my mother had brought with her from over the ocean, an assortment of superstitions.

"Don't step over the baby," she shrieked at one of us if we jumped over Harriet, as we tried to cross the crowded living room-bedroom floor where she played. "She won't grow."

I had to chew thread while my mother sewed a button on a dress I was wearing. It was much better to take the garment off to mend than to wear it. To counteract the danger of wearing the dress as it was sewed, I was required to chew thread.

"Why am I chewing this thread? What's going to happen if I don't?" I asked.

"I might sew up your brains. Then you could become a dummy," my mother answered.

"What if she already is one?" Esther asked.

My mother ignored all remarks and told me to keep chewing.

She knew how to contend with the Evil Eye. We had to use cunning to keep this demon of bad luck at bay. My parents followed a set of rules that were invaluable in handling the Evil Eye. The first rule was (1) Never call attention to yourself by bragging or boasting about your accomplishments, your good health, or your good luck. (2) Never speak glowingly about your family or your loved ones. (3) Never act in a proud or arrogant manner. (4) If someone else should praise your accomplishments or speak to you of your good fortune, make light of it, minimize it. Our parents rarely praised us or lauded our achievements in school. The Evil Eye was out there waiting to pounce on anyone who had it good.

My little sisters wore red ribbons around their wrists, and red ribbons were tied on the babies' cribs. Everyone knew that red was a lucky color. It warded off the Evil Eye. Another way of warding off the bad luck demon was uttering the phrase, "Kennehora zul nit shotten," and making a sound three times—a sound best described as a combination of blowing and spitting at the same time. As I grew older the whole concept of the Evil Eye seemed ridiculous to me, an absurd import from impoverished and uneducated parts of Europe. Many years later, to be on the safe side, I tied red ribbons on my babies' cribs. I never carried pictures of my children to whisk out for others to admire.

My father didn't argue about chewing thread when my mother sewed a button on his shirt while he wore it. He went along with the red ribbons and didn't step over any of us. Although he was steeped in tradition and myth from the Old World he was skeptical about them, and eager to know and experience the exciting changes taking place in the New World.

In Poland he had driven a horse and wagon. In America he bought a Chevy as soon as he had enough money. He quickly learned to drive, and he drove in a reckless and cavalier manner that made passengers cringe. Fearlessly, he careened around corners, turned suddenly without warning, and wove in and out of traffic. As soon as I was of age, he taught me his version of how to drive a car so I could deliver fish to our customers.

He kept a car for about ten years, rarely worrying about check ups, lubrication, or any kind of regular maintenance. Periodically strange noises would emanate from the car, or it might refuse to start or worse, to stop. It was only then that he took it for repair. As we grew older and more knowledgeable about cars, we insisted he try a regular schedule of maintenance. I suppose he felt a piece of machinery wasn't like a horse, upon whom he had once lavished so much attention.

His curiosity about space travel gave him the idea for a special project. During the fifties Pan American Airlines announced that a trip to the moon would someday be possible for their airline passengers. My father was excited by the idea and asked me if I would write a letter for him to Pan Am stating that he would like to be on the first commercial flight to the moon. Of course, I refused.

"It's foolish, Father. They'll think you're silly or worse. I don't want to be a party to this nonsense."

Not one to discourage easily, he approached Harriet, who wrote the letter for him. Incredulously, I read the reply he received a couple of weeks later. The company spokesperson wrote back that no trips were being planned for the immediate future, but my father would be put on a waiting list for the first trip. He was sent an identification card with his name and number on the waiting list. He was Number 407.

"You mean to tell me," I sputtered, "that there are 406 people who already want to be in on this harebrained ride?"

The company added that the cost would probably be out of this world. Jokingly, my father talked about the length of the trip and what he would need to take along.

It dawned on him that he would miss prayer services on this long journey to the moon. Immediately, he began recruiting his fellow worshippers to go along. His goal was nine men, who with himself, would make ten, a minyan. We were pleased when he reported that he had enlisted five easily. A little more cajoling and the number went up to seven. A firm promise to bring along plenty of Canadian Mist, and he had his minyan. Now it was possible to have communal worship services anywhere, and how fitting that they might all be closer to the heavens when they prayed. Good naturedly, the nine other men assured him that they would be ready to go whenever the trip became available. Such interests and activities enlivened his days, and my father enjoyed the laughter and discussion that ensued.

Not everyone was pleased about the proposed trip to the moon. It was with great surprise that my father listened to a tirade against him from the wife of one of the would-be travelers. She and her husband lived across the street above their hardware store. She was furious at my father and had run over to express her anger at him for involving her husband in the first moon trip.

"Mr. Schafer," she said shrilly, "I'm surprised at you. You know very well that we go to Florida every winter. Now that my husband promised you he'll go to the moon, what'll we do if it comes out in the winter? Just what are we supposed to do?"

He looked at her angry face. For once he was speechless. What in the world was there to say?

CHAPTER EIGHTEEN

Hollenbeck Street

I didn't want to move from Joseph Avenue, but everyone else in the family did. In late spring of 1941 my father purchased a large, attractive double house on Hollenbeck Street near Avenue A, a ten-minute walk from the store or four or five minutes by car. The owner who had had it built lost the house to the bank. It was up for sale. My father knew the owner and felt sorry about the foreclosure. "I won't buy it if you don't want I should," my father said to the owner.

"Go ahead, Sam. Someone else will buy it if you don't. I can't keep it. I'd be glad for you to get it."

The house had two large eight-room apartments. We moved into the downstairs apartment. The tenants, a family of four, lived upstairs. We had shiny hardwood floors, gum-wood trim, beveled-glass windows, and built-in bookcases with leaded glass doors. My father was proud of his acquisition. The house, spacious, surrounded by trees and grass, demonstrated his rise in the world. In his eyes Hollenbeck street embodied the better life for his family that he and my mother sought. With this move they were realizing their aspirations. He wanted us to be as happy as he was with our new home.

My sisters and I walked through it with him several times when it was empty, and he asked us what we wanted in the house. All of us said, "A fireplace." A gracious fireplace with a mantel over it was aristocratic. In so many books I had read, grand houses had a fireplace. I could picture myself curled up in a chair, reading in front of it. A real wood-burning fireplace could not be built in our living room, so the carpenter must have fashioned a make-believe fireplace that looked authentic to us. Above the fireplace he hammered into the wall an attractive piece of wood to serve as the mantel. We had make-believe logs that glowed red at the touch of a button. All of us enjoyed the effect. We put a large replica of an oil painting above the mantel. It was a still-life of magnolia blossoms arranged in a vase. In winters to come, my sisters and I gathered around the fireplace, and turned on the logs so they glowed red. I felt elegant as I sat gazing at the logs.

The rooms were big, and the kitchen almost had cupboards enough for all the sets of dishes my mother had—milchig and fleishig for every day as well as milchig and fleishig for Passover. Still, some of the pots, pans, and utensils had to go in the basement. Even with four bedrooms, two of us had to share a room until Marcia married and moved out. There were closets in every bedroom and a closet in the entry hall for coats. The space for living and for storage amazed us. One closet even had a door with a full-length mirror on it. It fascinated me, and I spent time talking to my image in the mirror.

My father hired a painter to give every room a fresh coat, and allowed us to help choose the colors. Esther liked all shades of pink, and enlisted our influence in securing a promise to paint the bathroom hot pink. Once it was done, the bathroom vibrated and pulsed with the bright color. It was hard for me to see what I really looked like when I gazed in the bathroom mirror. My face appeared bright pink. Even if I was pale or slightly sick, even deathly ill, I would only have to look in the bathroom mirror to feel better. When I had the flu it was hard to believe I was as sick as I felt because I had such a healthy glow. We all appeared amazingly healthy until we changed the color of the bathroom walls.

Outside of the house, to keep the garbage cans hidden from sight, there was a small brick shed in the backyard. And what a backyard it was. Our double house on a modest city street was built on a huge, deep lot that took up almost an entire city block. We had never had a backyard before, not with grass, trees, shrubs, and flower beds. It felt as if we had moved to a park. For the first time I heard birds twittering early in the morning outside my bedroom window. I enjoyed hearing the birds, but I missed the sounds of traffic.

It was a traumatic change for me—a street without stores. Only houses with front yards and back yards lined the street. The front yards were small, but they had grass all over. There were trees along the curb, birds flew about—birds I had only seen in picture books. I missed the dozens of people walking along the sidewalk, shopping and visiting. I missed the clang of the trolley, the library across the street, the creamery and the drugstore on either side of us. I liked being in the middle of all the bustle and activity. I missed everything familiar. I didn't want to be in what I thought was the countryside—with no stores right next to us.

I missed my neighborhood and my school where my teachers thought I was smart, and where everybody knew me. I liked everyone asking me hard questions. In my new school the boys and girls looked different. They dressed better, and they all seemed smart. I eventually found that most of their parents spoke better English than the parents of my old friends.

I heard one of my new classmates whisper to the person next to her, "Ruth's father has a fish market on Joseph Avenue. She probably smells like a fish."

I knew this snobby person's family had a shop on East Avenue, an elegant shop on an elegant street. It wasn't very nice to be a snob, so I told myself not to pay attention to her, but I was unhappy for months, and cried myself to sleep many nights. It took me a long time to get over growing up on Joseph Avenue. I wonder if I ever did.

My father now had a huge expanse of grass (our backyard) that needed to be cut. He acquired a small hand mower that worked well, but it took hours to complete the job of cutting the lawn. In winter, it took hours and prodigious energy to shovel the snow from the front and side door, as well as the driveway and along the walkway to the doors. He decided not to shovel the whole driveway to get to the garage, which was at the back of the yard. He kept his new Chevy just a little way into the driveway close to the street. The car never knew the protection of a garage in the winter. Every morning my father had to scrape the car windows clear of ice, and with an old broom he swept the snow from its top and sides.

We began to hold family picnics in our backyard in the summer, inviting aunts, uncles, and cousins. We had by far the largest piece of land of anyone. My parents bought lawn chairs, a hammock, and a table to better enjoy their outdoor life. We played croquet and badminton in the yard. My mother planted flowers beds. Even on Joseph Avenue she had tried to plant pansies in a little, tiny postage stamp of earth. Now she could plant roses, all kinds of border plants along the walk to the house, and of course, more of her favorite pansies. We even planted vegetables during World War II, our victory garden. A big chestnut tree next to the shed dropped spiky burrs every fall.

When we moved to Hollenbeck Street in 1941, we still came to help my father, but without the buzzer to call us downstairs, we were not so much at his beck and call. He used to telephone us instead, urging us to get over to the store as quickly as possible. With business improving, my father needed more help than the family could provide. He started to hire people. Ignatz, who spoke only Polish, could talk to no one but my father. Ignatz mostly cleaned fish or swept the floor. A small, wizened little man, he worked in the store for years. Trying to figure out his age was useless. He might have been 40 or possibly 70. None of us knew if he had friends or a family. He rolled his own cigarettes, taking a small pouch of tobacco from his pocket and tapping some of its contents into a square of thin paper. He then he rolled the paper up to form a cigarette I expected the whole thing to come apart in his mouth, but it never did.

My father hired Mr. Menton to deliver fish orders. He was short, round, and friendly. He rode a motorcycle on his rounds, and Schafer's Fish Market was, no doubt, the only store that could claim orders would be delivered by motorcycle. Mr. Menton put the orders in his sidecar. He carried a black pouch with a long black strap and a metal clasp slung over his shoulder and chest in which to put the money he collected. He wore a black visored cap and looked somewhat dashing, racing off to deliver fish on his motorcycle.

One of the men my father hired was a refugee who had no skills and had recently come to this country. My father taught him to clean fish and to understand how to run a business. He was generous in giving his time, and was shocked when his employee left without notice two days before Passover, the busiest time of the year. The whole family put in extra time to help make up for it.

As soon as I turned sixteen my father taught me to drive a car so I could deliver fish orders, too. Mr. Menton had, by then, probably gone on to a more lucrative job, and my father needed someone to get the orders out. He gave me driving lessons whenever he had a few extra minutes to spare. Later in life I had to unlearn much of what he taught me about driving. Most of our customers were not far away—Gladys Street, Conkey Avenue, Buchan Park, Vienna Street, Dorbeth Road— all streets I knew. I rarely drove for pleasure. I took a bus if I had to go somewhere.

Our move from Joseph Avenue and the hiring of help signaled a slow shift away from our intense involvement in the store. I had time to make new friends, and after a while I came to love our house on Hollenbeck Street. My sisters and I brought our friends over often, and sometimes we had parties at our house. When I was old enough to go out on dates, I occasionally sat in the backyard with a beau.

One summer night I had a date that ended early. I bid goodnight to my escort on our front steps, and after he left I found the house doors locked. My parents and younger sisters had probably gone out for a rare ride together, maybe to get ice cream. Because it was so warm and pleasant, I lay down on the hammock and gazed at the sky. The night was dark, and I looked at the stars, trying to trace the constellations. It was a sky that was not visible on Joseph Avenue.

The Chevy soon rolled up the driveway and into the garage. I heard my parents and sisters get out of the car, talking and laughing as they walked toward the house. I got up from the hammock and stood waiting for them. My father stopped. All talking and laughing ceased when they saw me standing. I heard my father say in a low voice, "Stay back, Kate, with the children."

His hands clenched into fists. He walked slowly and menacingly toward me—all five feet four inches of his stocky frame tensed and ready to fight. "Who are you? What do you want?" he asked as he advanced.

He couldn't see me well enough to make out who it was. "Father, it's only me. I got home early and couldn't get in," I said.

I could almost hear the exhalation of everybody's breath. My father unclenched his fists, and his whole body relaxed. We all started to laugh. Later, I thought about his determination to protect his family against an unknown assailant. Strong as he was, he knew nothing about fighting. It had been instinctive in him to step forward, to guard my mother and sisters from perceived harm. The one time he had been physically attacked and left for dead, he pretended to his assailant that he was unconscious before he had actually lapsed into unconsciousness. He had not fought back. In his hospital room and later, he sometimes wondered if he could have saved his eyesight by fighting off his attacker.

"Father, you said that man was young and big and strong-looking. He might have killed you for sure if you tried to hit him or strike out. You did the right thing to save your life. He thought you were a dead man when he ran out," I answered.

My reassurances could not stop his replaying the scene in his mind. For a long time he had nightmares. He called out and screamed. When he was awakened, he invariably was upset, almost breathless. "I was fighting with that man. I was punching him," he said each time.

CHAPTER NINETEEN

War

The earth-shaking events of the world did not seem to have a great impact on my life. World War II must have been of grave concern to my parents. They both had many family members still in Poland, but they didn't talk about it. They listened to the radio, sitting with their bodies perched forward on chairs. They gave the radio broadcasts their full attention. We heard Walter Winchell and his rapid fire delivery. He opened his news program with, "Good evening, ladies and gentlemen, and all the ships at sea." He spoke rapidly, and I think I remember the staccato sound of a telegraph punctuating his remarks.

Edward R. Murrow was more to my liking. He had a way of saying, "This is London," when he started his news program that was a portent of dramatic events to come. My parents also read the daily *Forward,* and they must have discussed the war with their friends and our relatives. My first cousin, Bernie Oratz, was a soldier. Our upstairs neighbor, Jack Sherman, was in the army, but as far as I was concerned the fighting was too far away to concern me. Most of my ideas of the war came from the movies. Just as I watched the screen to find out how "Americans" were supposed to talk and behave, I now sat in the darkened theater and watched what the Hollywood film industry showed us of the terrors of war. Explosions in the trenches, wounded soldiers, gunfire, submarine warfare, bombs falling, buildings crumbling, Japanese suicide attacks, hungry civilians—the suffering and waste of war were revealed, but I did not despair. The Good always won. American soldiers like John Wayne, Tyrone Power, Randolph Scott were brave. I knew the American soldier was strong and would be victorious. When a lone American was left to defend a stronghold against overwhelming odds, he would either be rescued at the last minute, wipe out the enemy, or go down fighting, a hero, his death vindicated by all that he had accomplished.

Beautiful, brave women in the movies were role models to me. I wanted to be like Lana Turner or Esther Williams, so beautiful and patriotic. They played heroic women who joined the service. Not only did they don uniforms to serve their country, they even found romance. Claudette Colbert saved lives as an army nurse, even as she struggled with her own personal problems. I told my mother that if I were older, I would join the WAACs or the WAVEs. She became agitated and said, "Nice girls don't join the Army or Navy." I argued with her, but not with much spirit, because I was too young, anyway. I couldn't figure out what was not nice about helping the war effort, and she could not explain.

Most of the war movies were full of action and violence. I avoided them as much as possible, but there were so many of them that some weeks that was all that was showing at the RKO Palace, the Loew's, or the Paramount. My girlfriend, Joyce, and I decided to see *The Sullivans.* Maybe we thought it was better than the other movies that were showing. Perhaps we thought it would not be too upsetting, and at first we seemed to have been right. We saw the five little Sullivan boys as children, growing up in a loving family, getting into scrapes. They were all such nice boys, and they were funny. We laughed at some of their misadventures. They came of age during the war, and they all wanted to join the Navy and stay together during the conflict. We were not prepared to have them all perish when their ship went down. I stared at the screen not comprehending at first. Then when I understood the terrible tragedy, I started to sob, and so did Joyce. When the naval representative came and knocked on the Sullivan family door, I wanted to look away. Mrs. Sullivan knew, when she saw the serious face of the messenger, that something was wrong. She asked haltingly, "Which one?" I couldn't bear to listen. What were Joyce and I doing in this movie theater? Why were we here watching? I had my hands over my face, but I looked between my fingers. Mrs. Sullivan was waiting for an answer to her question. When the messenger said, "All of them," Joyce and I were overcome with emotion. At the end of the movie we got up silently, unable to speak. We went outside into the daylight, our hearts too heavy to comfort each other. We took the bus home without saying a word.

Looking back I am shocked at my lack of awareness of my own aunts, uncles and cousins who were probably in concentration camps. What became of them? How is it I did not even know of them? My father had no pictures of any of the Schafers. After the war I found a few old pictures of my mother's family. One of the pictures taken when Uncle Yitzrak Oratz went back to visit the family in the late twenties, showed my mother's parents, her sisters, their husbands, and their little children. My cousins were young. Curling dark hair framed small serious faces. One of my little girl cousins stood next to her grandfather, her hand resting on his knee. A boy of four or five sat on the floor with a mischievous half smile on his face. Another cousin, who was probably my age, wore a dress with a big collar and a bow in her hair. She looked out at me. I never found out what happened to any of them

Because the movies brought the war to my consciousness, I wanted to do something useful. Children in other places in our country directly helped the war effort. I read about them in *Current Events*, a newspaper to which all the seventh graders subscribed. Campfire Girls in one city placed over one hundred collection cans in their town so patriotic citizens could drop old keys in them. The Campfire Girls collected the full cans and turned them in for scrap.

In North Adams, Massachusetts, the Junior Red Cross staged a patching party in which members collected patches to mend work socks to make them last longer. They also darned torn socks.

School children in Seattle made games for our men in the armed forces—checker sets, chess sets, and Chinese checkers. I read that in our own hometown, a five-year-old Junior Commando, by tirelessly scouring his neighborhood, single-handedly (unless you count his mother) collected an estimated 500 pounds of outworn kitchen utensils, broken tools, discarded lengths of steel pipes and rusty bed springs. Doubtless other outworn and outmoded objects were also dragged home in his little wagon to be turned over to the scrap-iron drive.

The only memory I have of doing something constructive is attending War Bond assemblies in school. Famous movie stars came to our schools to talk about why we should buy bonds. Naturally, we had to ask our parents ahead of time what, if anything, we could buy. When Franchot Tone came to our school I cajoled my parents into allowing me to buy a twenty-five dollar bond. Dorothy Lamour was another big fund-raiser.

My family also tried to plant a victory garden. We now had our block-long backyard, and with much effort by my father we converted a small plot of grass into a vegetable garden. I was an indifferent gardener and helped when necessary. I do not recall that we ever had much of a crop.

My biggest contribution to the war effort was helping my father count the ration books in the store. Fish was not rationed, but our groceries were. Everybody had to do with less. Items such as ketchup, sugar, butter; and some canned goods required ration stamps. Blue stamps were for canned food and red stamps were for meat, butter, and fats. The government issued ration books good for 52 weeks. The idea was to keep inflation down and to spread scarce food evenly throughout the population. My father told me he was never part of the black market, but his accounting system of stamps and ration books was far from precise. I remember government inspectors coming into the store admonishing my father that his record keeping was very poor, and he had to do better. An inspector told him, "You can't give anybody anything that's rationed without getting the necessary stamps."

My father argued, "What if a man comes in and says he needs more food for his children? What would you do? Wouldn't you give him what he needs?" Although inspectors came in from time to time, my father continued in his belief that it was his duty to help parents feed their children whether they had the right number of stamps or not. Perhaps his years of hunger and want had left an indelible mark on him, for all his life he threw caution to the winds to help anyone who needed food.

The war ended during the week of my fifteenth birthday. My parents and my sisters took me to see a movie to make the day extra special. That we were in a movie theater together was itself a special event. We had heard on the radio that the end was near, but we actually saw the celebrations of victory in the movie theater. Probably my parents had wanted to see news of the end of the war, too. Everyone in the theater clapped, cheered, and stamped their feet when the RKO Pathe News showed our boys in uniform being feted in the streets of whatever towns they liberated. I was moved by the scenes of jubilation. The war was finally over.

CHAPTER TWENTY

Land of Enchantment

I hugged my parents and sisters one more time. "Bye, Mama, don't cry. Father, you don't need to worry about me." Then I turned to board the Empire State Express. The train started to pull away. I kept waving until I couldn't see any of them.

I sat back, still amazed that I was on my way to New Mexico. Why did they let me go so far from their watchful eyes? I'd never even been to summer camp or rarely eaten anywhere but my parents' kitchen.

The most compelling reason was my health, a topic not talked about in our home. For years I had suffered from severe allergies and chronic sinus. I sounded as though I had a bad cold or terrible hay fever all year. I could not breathe through my nose, so my throat was always dry, and I often had a dull headache. Still I didn't let it stop me from participating in activities at school, with friends or at the store. I rarely mentioned my sinus problems to anyone because such a physical failing was considered by my parents to be a detriment to a girl's marriage prospects.

"Maybe a hot dry, climate will help your daughter," the doctor said. I had graduated high school and was toying with the idea of college. The doctor suggested Arizona or New Mexico. In July I half-heartedly applied to both state universities, thinking it was too late to get in and, my parents wouldn't let me go anyway. I received an acceptance from the University of New Mexico within a short time, and I was soon packing my new foot locker in a daze at this turn of events.

The most important factor of all, I think, was that they trusted me.

"You'll meet wolves out there," my father had said

"I know how to handle wolves," I answered with confidence. He said later that he made up his mind then, that I could be trusted so far away from home. I tried to live up to that trust.

The landscape in New Mexico was so different from that of New York. I loved the desert, the mesa, the Sandia mountains that rose close by. The students looked different—Mexicans, Indians, plain whites, and mixtures of all the cultures. It was exciting.

My first stop was the freshman dorm, Bandelier Hall, an adobe building. Two girls and I shared a small room, none of us knowing anyone else. I wondered if we would like each other. I was incredibly fortunate. We became the best of friends, I knew I was lucky to have two such compatible and lovely roommates. Someone in our hall commented that the three of us got along beautifully even though we represented three major religions, rural and urban backgrounds, southwestern and northeastern cultures. Colleen was Protestant from a small community not far from Albuquerque, Eleanor was Catholic from San Antonio, and I from New York state with my Jewish We-just-got-off-the-boat background. Eleanor and Colleen both spoke with a southern drawl. Their speech was pleasing to my ear. I enjoyed hearing all the different speech patterns of my classmates—from the native Americans to those from New York City.

I loved everything about that freshman year—even the classes. My father always said, "Whatever you're doing, do your best." I studied hard so my grades were good and getting better. It was fun talking to my classmates and finding out where they came from and what they were planning to be. I could meet and greet everyone easily, probably from my experiences with customers. I was elected president of my dorm. I felt "popular," a strange feeling that was new and heady. I could concentrate on my studies and on my social life without the distractions of the fish market, or the obligations of family. It was liberating.

Sometimes I tried to cheer up homesick classmates who were

crying. "Where are you from?" I usually asked. Many of the students were from New Mexico, not far from their hometown. I didn't seem to find the time to be homesick because everything was new and different Still, I was mindful of my parents' teachings. That year I became a vegetarian, because I refused to eat all non-kosher meat. I did eat fish with scales whenever it was served. At Passover, the Aranow family, who had Rochester roots, invited me for the seders, where I ate heartily.

Periodically my parents sent me food. Once they sent me a whole boiled chicken, but I had no place to keep it. I managed to eat a drumstick before I put the package in my dresser drawer next to my sweaters. I couldn't find anyone to share it with. There was no one in the dorm who wanted some plain boiled chicken. When I looked at the chicken two days later it was already turning green. I asked my parents to not send any more cooked chicken. Although most of the students complained about the cafeteria food, I enjoyed what I ate. I had always enjoyed institutional food.

Another one of my parents' strictures was that I date only boys of our faith. I was prepared to limit my dating activity. To my surprise there were dozens of Jewish young men who had come to this hot dry state because of a respiratory ailment. I joined Hillel and met dozens. My social life improved, but my sinus problems had not improved. Being unable to breathe through my nose meant that long kisses were out of the question. When necessary I explained the need for short kisses and found that honesty was the best policy.

I relished the time I spent with my roommates and all the friends I had made. In spring I met a tall, dark, and handsome graduate student. He asked me to the spring ball. That evening the gym was festooned with balloons and streamers. We danced and laughed, and as I looked up at him there flashed in my mind the movie I had seen years before of such a gym festooned with balloons and streamers. How I had longed to be a part of such a happy carefree life. Now I was living my dream.

When I said goodbye in June, I had hoped that I might be coming back. But I never returned. My parents felt it was pointless to let me return if the climate had not helped my sinus trouble. No matter how much I pleaded or argued they said I should finish college at the University of Rochester. For months I wept. I walked around sullen and silent. I was homesick for New Mexico, for the people I cared about there. Living at home and. going to the U of R was like going to high school. But one day I made a conscious decision to stop crying. I told myself that my parents were paying for a valuable education, and they wanted me home to help them. I needed to make new friends and appreciate what I had. So I put the past year away and immersed myself in the present. Eventually I met a tall, dark, handsome musician and married him.

When I think of my freshman year, I recall scenes from a past that would have lead to a different life. I cannot know what kind of person I would have become, but I know I would not have returned to Rochester to live. There was in that landscape and that lifestyle an openness and freedom that lifted my spirits and showed me another world. But if I had remained there, I would not have known the closeness and love of my family life here or the marriage and children that I cherish.

The memories of the year in New Mexico shimmer and glow with a beauty all their own—a reminder that our lives can take many different paths.

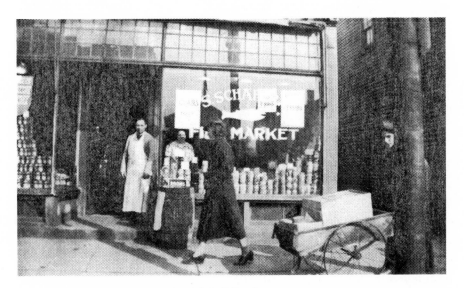

Fish Market

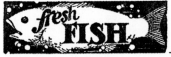

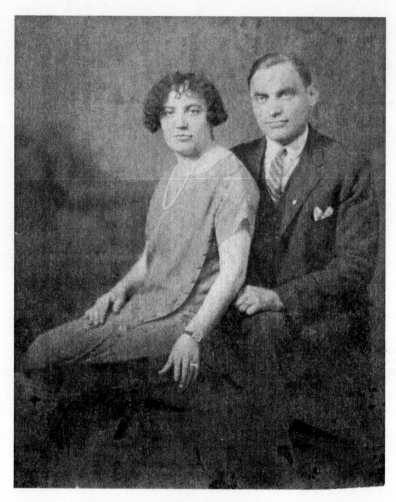

Engagement

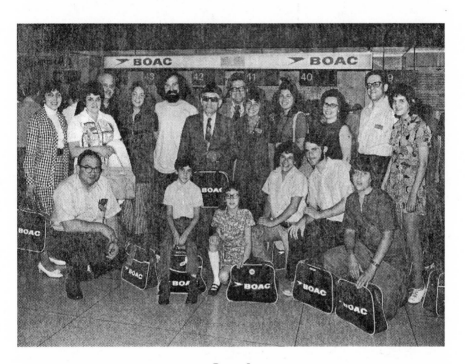

Israel

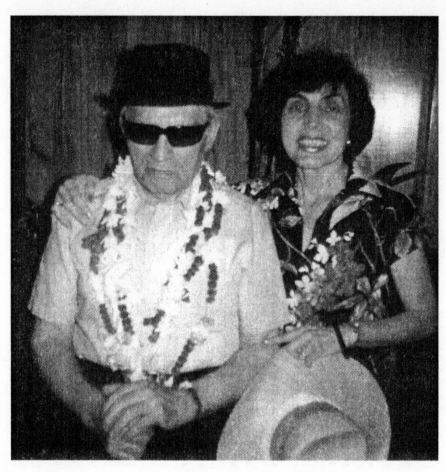

Sam and Ruth

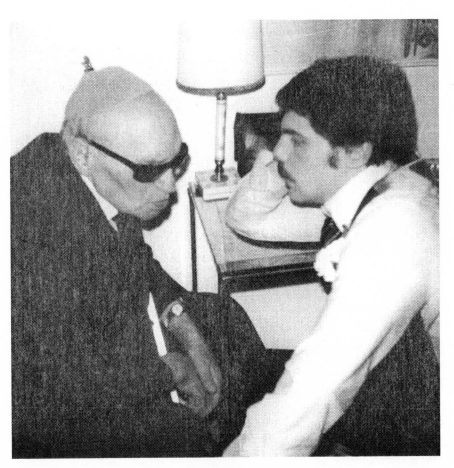

Sam and Paul

CHAPTER TWENTY-ONE

Mother

I didn't know her very well because we never talked together much, not about anything that mattered. She was my mother. She took good care of my sisters and me, combing my hair and making sausage curls, cooking our meals, and cleaning the house, helping my father in the store. She didn't have time to talk to me. How could she? Where did she find the time to assemble meals from fresh ingredients, follow all the time-consuming rituals of our religion, especially for the holidays and the Sabbath, take care of us four girls, and still clean and wrap fish in the store? She worked from early in the morning until late at night without a break, going from the house to the store and back. I couldn't imagine my life without her. She died when she was 57 years old, and I never had time to talk to her about herself. I was married by then and had two very young children. She had already had a couple of heart attacks and could not help me with the children. I could not afford a babysitter, had no car, and therefore could not visit her during the day.

If I'd only known how little time remained to us I would have somehow tried to see her more often, spent time paying attention, talking to her, listening to her, but I was too busy, and time ran out. I learned from my mistake. My father lived much longer. I had more time to get to know him. I talked to him and listened. I spent time paying attention.

As a young child I never saw my parents argue. If they voiced disagreement it must have been late at night or somewhere out of our sight. One time I saw my mother upset. I was five or six years old, and I was playing alone in the "backyard" behind the store. It was a small area of cement and a tiny patch of grass. Our three-car garage took up the rest of the space. Originally the garage had been a barn. The hayloft was still there. Sometimes I climbed up the wooden steps that led to the loft, and looked at the empty space. I was afraid to venture into the unused loft itself because some of the floorboards were missing or broken, but down in the yard I played for many hours. In the midst of my playing that day, my mother came out and sat down on the high back step. There were no clothes or diapers hanging out to dry, so I did not have to avoid a line full of flapping aprons or underwear. She did not talk to me or watch what I was doing. I had never seen her sit idly in the middle of the day. She was always doing something. She never stopped cleaning, cooking, watching over us, or working in the store. I knew something was wrong. I think I asked her if she felt all right. She must have said yes, but her eyes were shiny with unshed tears. I can still remember her sitting there quietly, trying to regain her composure. When I think of it now, it fills me with a great sadness. I wish I had known how to make her feel better. If I had been older I might have asked her why she felt sad. I could have asked her what she would like to change, what would make her happier.

My father seemed to make the big decisions—where we lived and how we lived. Still, I knew my mother wielded great power over him. He wanted her love and approval for his hard work and accomplishments. She could not give her approval. I realize now that she did not like his being in business. She did not believe in his philosophy of volume buying, of plowing profits back into the business. They argued about it openly when we were older. She did not want to be involved in any real-estate ventures. She would have preferred to live in a single house, not a double. He did quell his interest in real estate investing for her sake. As we grew older, they argued more. It was always about the business, the hours he spent in it, the time it took away from the family, the money he put into it.

His manner of arguing was to say what he wanted, or what course of action he wanted to take, and if he didn't get his way or if my mother refused to agree with him, he would sulk. All of us would get the silent treatment. He was usually talkative, so his withdrawal was noticeable. The silence might last several days. It was upsetting to everyone. In the end problems were resolved—his way.

Whatever her feelings were, my mother always worked hard. When she had first come to this country as a young woman of about twenty she found a job making lapels or buttonholes at a large clothing factory, Hickey-Freeman. She had snapshots taken at that time showing her with other young women, laughing and enjoying the camaraderie of her colleagues. A formal picture taken at a studio shows her with her sister and a girlfriend, all wearing party dresses. My mother's dress was black with a pattern of beads all the way down the front. The beads were small and black and they shone. It was a beautiful dress. I saw it hanging in my mother's closet for years, but I never saw her in it. She probably had no place to wear it. Once married there were no parties, light hearted get-togethers, or social activities outside of the family. I have a beaded bag of hers from those party days. I could tell she enjoyed beautiful things and that she liked being with people.

When she married it seemed that she had exchanged the life of a single, smiling, working girl for an arduous life as my father's helpmate. Most often she wore a big white apron sprinkled with fish scales or the blood of fish she had decapitated. She was a working mother who deftly juggled all her tasks from nursing and diapering babies, cooking, baking, and housecleaning to waiting on customers and cleaning fish for them.

She died after suffering a fourth heart attack. My baby daughter, Judy, was a year old, and my son, David, was two. I found out she was back in the hospital when my sister, Marcia, late one afternoon, called to tell me.

"Mother's heart is acting up again. She's at Strong."

"I'll see her after supper," I told Marcia. "I've got to feed the kids first.

After supper was too late. When I asked for my mother's room number, the nurse took me aside. "Your mother just died. I'm very sorry, but we couldn't do anything to save her," the nurse said.

I sat there. If I'd come when Marcia called me I would have seen her, maybe talked to her. I would have been with her. I could have told her I loved her. She had argued with me a few days before, and there was still a coolness between us. I never forgave myself for not being there.

When my father arrived soon after, my sisters and I surrounded him and told him of her death. He looked dazed.

"Are they sure? Can't they do something? Can't they put in her a new heart?"

This was 1959. We didn't know about heart transplants. I thought my father was crazed with grief to make such an absurd suggestion.

After the formal period of mourning was over, my father lived alone for a while on Hollenbeck Street. Two years after my mother's death the Star Super Market bought the house because they wanted the land. To replace the double on Hollenbeck Street, he bought a double house a block away from Dan and me and lived in one side. Moving was apparently not too difficult for my father, but breaking up the last home my parents had lived in together was very hard for me. It held so many memories of our growing up years.

I came to help pack the objects that he didn't want the movers to take. We had a month or more to remove everything. The house was empty, and I took my time looking at the pieces that reminded me of my mother. I found a pretty green glass juicer that she had used before the advent of frozen orange juice. Every morning she would cut the oranges in half. She fit one half over the hump of the juicer and turned the orange back and forth. The pits and some fiber would fall into the juice. Sometimes she strained the juice, but I preferred it with the bits and pieces. Freshly squeezed orange juice was a part of our daily breakfast, and so much better than canned orange juice, with its somewhat strange taste. Marcia said it tasted "tinny," but when oranges were out of season we drank it.

So much of my mother's life was centered in the kitchen. She made most of our meals from scratch. I still have a wooden rolling pin that she used, a long narrow wooden cylinder that tapers at the ends. She made challah and puter kuchen fairly often, rolling the dough and sprinkling flour on the rolling pin and table as she worked. The kuchen was made of a sweet dough that took hours to rise. She pulled apart handfuls of dough from the tub, shaped them, and filled them with blueberries (yagedes). She decorated each little mound of dough with curlicues and dots of dough because she wanted them to look nice. Every available counter space in the kitchen and pantry was lined with pans of kuchen rising for the final time before they were put into the oven. The aroma as they baked filled the house. Now I wish I had her recipe. They were the best blueberry kuchens in the world.

She knew little about American-style cuisine. We told her about spaghetti. "It's good American food, Mama, and it's kosher." We explained that they were noodles, not flat ones like the ones we had in chicken soup, but round. They were always in a red sauce. "Can't we have it for supper tomorrow?" Esther asked. Marcia ran down to the store and brought up a box. We followed the cooking directions on the box. My mother took out a big aluminum colander and drained the spaghetti.

"The box says to use your favorite tomato sauce," I reported. "We can use ketchup. It's just like tomato sauce." We were pleased to have American food. I use her aluminum colander now.

Before the movers came to Hollenbeck Street to take the furniture to my father's new home, I went into the backyard and dug up some flowers to take with us. Whenever I see pansies I think of my mother. She loved flowers, and every year she planted them. Even when we lived on Joseph Avenue she filled the narrow strip of soil with pansies. Such piquant faces they had, especially the yellow ones. The backyard on Joseph Avenue was mostly cement and brick, but when we moved to Hollenbeck Street we had a huge yard, and she could take a trowel and a little shovel and plant to her heart's content. She cut pieces from a rosebush in the yard and planted them in a row, covering them with upside-down mayonnaise jars to protect the cuttings. Most of the roses grew.

One of my favorite possessions that belonged to my mother was a set of little square glasses in a glass holder. I think they came from Europe. She either brought the set with her or it was sent to her. I never knew how they were meant to be used or what they were. Almost everything in our house was bought when my parents were married or later. We had no family heirlooms or precious pieces with a history. The little glass set is the closest to an "old" family treasure. It sat in our china closet and was never used because we never knew what to do with it.

My mother and her sister, May, had come to this country with nothing except what they carried. Between them they had five dollars, according to an immigration list. They came alone leaving behind their parents, their friends, and their language. They had memories of hiding in their family's cellar as Russian soldiers ran through the village looking to pillage and rape. Uncle Abraham sponsored them, but when they arrived here they lived with their brother, Isadore, and his family for a short while.

In time my mother became engaged, but the engagement was broken off shortly before the wedding. I found an old picture in which half was cut off. "You cut somebody out of the picture. How come?" I asked.

She didn't answer and never spoke about it. My father supplied the information. He said it was a picture of my mother with her fiancé (he used the word "boyfriend"). She cut him out of the picture when the engagement ended. In the thin strip of photograph remaining, my mother appeared smiling and smartly dressed in a fur-trimmed wrap. I suppose she liked the way she looked in her fashionable outfit so much that she kept her half of the picture. She refused to talk about this part of her life.

"What happened, Mother? Why did you break your engagement?" one of us asked her every once in a while. My father told us, after she had died, that Uncle Abraham apparently was not going to give the "boyfriend" the promised dowry. Perhaps there had been a misunderstanding about the amount. Maybe there was another reason.

Whatever the cause, she remained silent, and we never heard from her lips the story behind the broken engagement. My father had wanted no dowry. For him it was love that mattered.

"Did you ever find out who this boyfriend was?" we asked him.

"Oh sure. I knew him. He had a business selling nuts. He was the nut man."

"What?" we all shrieked. We knew the nut store, and we knew the nut man.

"How could she even look at him?" we asked. "You're so much more handsome."

"I can't believe this," Harriet muttered, more to herself than us.

"Wasn't she lucky that didn't work out?" I said.

"We were all lucky," said Esther. It didn't even cross my mind that a nut store would have been so much easier to work in.

CHAPTER TWENTY-TWO

Mother and Mary

My mother rarely spent time with me alone. Once she took me with her to a movie, *May Time,* with Jeannette McDonald and Nelson Eddy. Although the story has faded from my memory, I know it was sad. When I was older she took me to see the Ballet Russe De Monte Carlo. Alone she went to an opera which was touring at that time. My father dropped her off at the Eastman Theater and picked her up after the performance. He stayed home to take care of us. They didn't go out together except to visit relatives.

Only one time do I remember my mother and father going out together. They went to a Yiddish-language show with Aunt May and Uncle David, who lived in the flat below ours. They left the three of us alone. My mother was pregnant with Harriet. Marcia was almost 12, and very mature. Perhaps a baby sitter could not be found, or maybe we said we didn't need a baby sitter. Our parents talked about who to call in an emergency, and what to do in every situation imaginable. Reassuring them all would be well with us, we sent them off. Esther fell asleep before they were down the stairs.

Not too long after they left I thought I heard footsteps on the stairs. Marcia didn't hear anything, but I frightened her.

"Let's lock the door," I suggested, "then no one can come in." Marcia took the big skeleton key and locked us in, but she couldn't get the key out. Although we couldn't move the key at all, we felt safer.

When our parents came home, they couldn't get in. They knocked on the door. "Open the door," my father said loudly through the door.

"We can't. The key won't turn," Marcia called back.

"Turn it to the left. It turns to the left," he told her. It didn't turn to the left.

"Try turning it to the right." It didn't turn to the right.

"Try harder," my father shouted. Marcia tried to turn it with all her might and broke the key in the lock. The top half was in her hand—the bottom remained in the lock. Esther woke up because of the loud shouting, and started to cry. My parents on the other side were upset, yelling for us to keep calm.

The noise had brought my aunt and uncle up the stairs to help. Uncle David, the self-proclaimed biblical scholar, knew absolutely nothing about things as mechanical as locks. My father who was probably a little more knowledgeable, did not know one end of a hammer from the other. I could hear them trying to figure out what to do. I was afraid we might never get out, and I wanted to cry, too.

All four of them were talking, interrupting each other, making suggestions.

"Call the police or the fire department," said Aunt May.

"Smash down the door," my uncle, our downstairs tenant, said.

"Let's try to take the door down without breaking it," my father, the landlord said. "We need to pull out the hinges."

They agreed, and a hiatus in their efforts ensued while my father went to get tools to implement their plan. In the meantime they kept telling Esther not to cry, assuring us we would get out. It took some time, but they finally pulled the hinges out, and my father placed the door against the wall. We were reunited with cries of joy and happiness more suitable to prisoners of war being rescued by a liberating army. I don't remember my parents going out together for years after that.

Most of my mother's time was spent caring for her four daughters, taking care of the house, and working with my father in the store. She washed clothes in the bathtub. My father, kneeling at the tub, helped her by scrubbing badly soiled items on a washboard. He wrung out the dripping laundry and helped hang it up outside. After baby Harriet was born, we acquired a Hoover washing machine and put away the washboard. The washing machine in the cellar had a wringer on it so the wet laundry could be squeezed dry. When we were older we all helped take the wet wash up the cellar stairs and outside to hang. In winter we hung the wash in the cellar, where it dried stiff in the cold air just as it did outside.

Added to all her ordinary everyday work were the tasks involved in observing the Jewish holidays. At Passover she soaped and wiped every surface. Cleaning all the cupboards, the refrigerator, and the stove were only part of the maelstrom of activity. All the holidays involved big meals, special foods, and long days at the synagogue.

Hiring a "girl" to help her at home enabled my mother to work in the store. Domestic help was relatively cheap. One of our best-loved baby sitters was Mrs. Gursky, whom I can barely remember. In my mind I see her rocking my little sister, Esther, in her arms. She was German, a grandmotherly woman. My mother trusted her completely. We missed Mrs. Gursky when she retired from baby sitting.

Then came Helen, who watched us several times a week. She also did some ironing, cleaning, and dusting. After a few months she told my mother she was leaving because she had found another job.

"I'm sorry to leave, Mrs. Schafer," she said, " but in my new job I get fifteen cents an hour, and I don't have to iron. There aren't so many children to watch, either." Maybe Helen expected my mother to offer her more money, but my mother only wished her luck in her new job.

In the summer months, the sweat rolled down our faces even if we sat motionless in our flat above the store. My father rented a cottage in Charlotte and sent my mother and us little girls to escape the stuffy, crowded flat. Jean, a pretty young woman, was willing to leave town when our whole family (except for my father) went to Charlotte. The way some people go to the French Riviera, we went to Charlotte on Lake Ontario. It took close to an hour to get there in our 1936 Chevy.

My father came down over the weekend, leaving Rochester Friday afternoon well before the Sabbath started. On Saturday he walked to a small synagogue in Summerville. Sunday morning he went back to the store alone. Jean stayed with us about two weeks to help my mother, but she left before the month was up, saying the work was too hard.

The most unforgettable person who helped my mother was Mary. She came with her own four children, who played with us. My big sister and I were old enough to help with our two younger sisters, but my mother's health was declining. Mary came once a week for twenty years to clean and iron for my mother. I grew up with Mary around and got used to her questions. She asked me about President Roosevelt. "Is he Jewish?"

"No, Mary," I said. "We've never had a Jewish president. Besides, Roosevelt isn't a Jewish name."

"Are you sure? I know it's not Eyetalian." Mary was Italian. "How about the guy who owns McCurdy's?" McCurdy's was a big department store. "He's Jewish isn't he?"

"He's not Jewish, either. I think that's a Scotch or Irish name."

"Oh, I thought the Jews owned all the stores."

"No, Mary, not all of them."

"Do you know why Negroes are black?" she asked. Mary was interested in people's origins

"'Why?" I dared myself to hear her answer.

"Because they're all born at night. White people are born in the daytime."

"Mary, that's not true. The time of day you're born has nothing to do with your color." I don't think she believed me.

She became a family retainer. When my mother died Mary asked if she could come to each of us. By then we were all married. I did not take up her offer until years later when I could afford some help and was going to graduate school. My children were already teenagers.

She continued her questions, turning her attention to the children. I entered the kitchen one morning just in time to hear her ask my fifteen year old son David, "Have you ever had a woman?" David was turning shades of red.

"Mary, we don't ask those kinds of questions."

She desisted from questioning him further, and turned her attention to me. Ruthie, does your husband beat you much?"

"Never."

"Never?" She stopped polishing the table.

"My mother told me that if a man raises his hand to me, I should leave and never come back."

"My Nick hits me when he's drunk. What about other women? Does he have any?"

"As far as I know my husband does not have any other woman." I was thinking that I should not work in the same room with her. I would go upstairs.

Mary was bitter about her husband's philandering. She had harsh words to say about Nick. "Let him go to his women," she ranted. "He likes them because they do whatever he wants in bed. Not me. I'm not going to do what he wants."

Frequently I chose not to be home when Mary came. When her husband died she telephoned me immediately after the funeral. "Ruthie, I stopped and bought a talking bird after I left the cemetery. I named him Nick after my husband. Do you want to hear him say something?"

"Sure, Mary. I'd love to hear him talk."

"Nikki, say something."

There was complete silence.

"C'mon, Nikki, say something to Ruthie."

Again silence.

"He was talking on the way home from the pet store," Mary said. She was exasperated. "C'mon ya dumb bird; say something." Nikki refused to talk. Apparently he was as perverse as his namesake.

Mary gave herself hourly pay raises. Without saying anything she came later and left earlier. As she aged I needed to pick her up and take her home. My sisters, who had managed to terminate her in a friendly way, asked why she still came. They felt she simply moved things around and stacked papers. I said she stacked papers neatly. The rooms looked better because the clutter was nicely arranged. Besides, Mary wanted to work. She loved making things clean. She had a sense of ownership over the tables and floors that she polished. "Ruthie, how do you like my kitchen floor? Doesn't it look beautiful?"

" Yes, it does, Mary. Nobody can get a floor as clean as you do." My answer was a lie. Her work was now slipshod, but I did not know how to end our working relationship gracefully. Then we had a falling out. She had been arriving late and leaving before the time agreed. She called me on the phone and asked for more money. I refused. She became angry and abusive.

"Mary, there's no use talking anymore. We'll say things we're going to be sorry about. I'll say goodbye." I gently put the phone down. About a month later she called back to say she was sorry we had argued. She missed me. She would come back at the same pay rate. I told her that Dan was retiring, and together we planned to do our work, but that if I ever needed help I would be sure to call her. Thus our long relationship ended on a friendly note. Sometimes when I look around at the disarray in our house I think of Mary and how well she stacked papers and rearranged clutter.

* * *

My mother's death wrought a sea change in our family. When she died my father was not quite sixty. Four months before her death, Harriet, the youngest, had married and moved out. My father was alone, but he was healthy and strong and financially secure. In time he could have found another wife. He preferred to live alone, ignoring overtures from widow ladies who brought soup and other enticements to the store for him.

"I made for you a honey cake, Mr. Schafer. You'll like it." She was a pleasant woman who smiled sweetly as she handed him the cake. He thanked her, took it home, and made a face when he took a bite. He told me, "It 's so dry it tastes like sand."

When customers asked why he didn't marry, he often laughed and said, "I'm happy the way I am. My family keeps me busy."

Immediately after our mother's funeral we four sisters had convened to talk about what to do for him. He was independent and insisted on remaining in his own home. One thing we knew; we had to make sure he had Sabbath dinner on Friday night and Saturday's meal after morning services. That was an absolute—the one immutable constant in his changed world. All of us decided to eat the Sabbath and holiday meals with him at his house because he would not drive to us on the Sabbath or the holidays. We planned to share in the making of the meals. No matter what our personal beliefs, we made every effort to carry on the family traditions that meant so much to him, and that gave us the impetus for our frequent family gatherings.

We learned to cooperate, to accommodate, to work through our differences as we planned how to share every occasion. Who would buy the food for the meals? What kind of menu would we make within the limits of our restrictions? Who would cook or bake or roast the food? How could we arrange our schedules to take turns for all the responsibilities? My mother's death provided the catalyst that brought us closer together. Our family's situation created a kind of laboratory in which we learned to meet the problems we faced, in which we tried to figure out what worked and what created tensions. We struggled to meet the challenges and in so doing unknowingly laid the groundwork for dealing with the even greater crisis of his blindness that was still many years away.

CHAPTER TWENTY-THREE

Real Estate

I was too young to help my father in his landlord role when we lived above the fish market. That building also housed three apartments. He must have been proud that he was able to purchase 584 Joseph Avenue. Ownership conferred upon him a feeling of accomplishment, a validation of his growing success as a merchant, and a sense of control over his life. It was when we moved into our double house on Hollenbeck Street that I began to realize some of the responsibilities of having tenants. We lived downstairs, and a family of four lived upstairs. I saw that my father handled all complaints with equanimity, but my mother did not enjoy the role of landlady and wanted no part of it.

My father believed that his money could grow faster invested in real estate. My mother tried to discourage my father from buying more property. It was bad enough for her to be living in a double house. She did not want to hear about plumbing problems or deal with tenants. She complained to my father that she did not like to hear people walking overhead. He said, "The tenants can't sit still all day—they haf to keep moving around." My parents' differing beliefs were a source of contention between them. I agreed with my father. I was interested in his ideas of growing money, but I tried to placate my mother. For her sake, he curbed his interest in buying real estate and stopped talking about it. Throughout her life she never changed her mind about a bank savings account being the best place to put her money.

It was a few years after her death in 1959 that my father began to pursue his vision of becoming a property owner on a larger scale. "I want to buy an apartment building," he said to me.

"You don't know anything about it, and neither do I."

"It's like having a double house, only you make more money. I'll start to look. You'll go with me, and we'll find one."

I heard the excitement in his voice. His face was animated. His blue eyes were alive with the anticipation of a search. I caught the excitement. I shared his vision, but I was afraid, too. We didn't know very much. That didn't seem to worry him.

"Let's not get a big place. Let's start small," I said.

I accompanied him on his first search expeditions, leaving the children with Dan. Nothing appealed to us. We kept looking at small apartment houses, climbing stairs, gazing at roofs, trudging through narrow hallways, turning on faucets, staring at furnaces.

One Sunday afternoon we had just gone through a building with small rooms and a very steep staircase. My father wasn't happy. I could tell by his expression.

"Let's keep moving," he advised Marvin, our agent. "Time is money, and we're not accomplishing anything standing here."

"I think this place might have potential, Sam," said Marvin.

"I don't like it. It doesn't appeal. Didn't anything new come on the market this week?"

Marvin took us to the next building on his list. It was old, had twelve units, half of which were vacant, and it needed repairs of all kinds.

"It's too big for us isn't it, Father?" I asked. "We can't handle twelve units."

"It's not too big," he answered.

The apartments had high ceilings, and were bright, with sunlight streaming through the long windows. I looked at my father. He was happy. I could tell by his expression, although he was good at disguising his pleasure. He did not want Marvin to see his avid interest.

"This isn't bad," he said noncommittally. "I like the neighborhood."

The area was becoming popular. Young people were moving into the trendy Park Avenue section, a neighborhood of shops, boutiques, restaurants, cafes, outdoor eating establishments and a myriad of services, such as dry cleaners, banks, and drugstores, along with delicatessens, small food markets and avant-garde clothing stores. He bought the building, and thus began his venture into the realm of high finance, as he liked to think of it.

"First, all the empty apartments we have to rent," father said.

That became the top priority on my agenda. I did all the legwork and the paperwork, Harriet took care of the books. My telephone number went into the newspaper. I stayed home so I could answer the phone and set up appointments. I ran back and forth to the building at all hours to show it to prospective renters. It took me time to realize that I could arrange viewing times that would suit me as well as the viewer.

In order to comply with the building codes and to make the building more attractive, I called and met with plumbers, electricians, painters, carpenters, plasterers and roofers. To find them I used my father's contacts among his customers. They were a good resource. If that failed I looked in the yellow pages. We had bought the building without a certificate of occupancy in exchange for a reduction in the selling price. We were required to make the necessary repairs within a specified time. I hurried to accomplish this. At the same time, I collected rents, knocked on doors of late paying tenants, and took care of complaints. Whenever I walked into the building I was met by tenants who were having problems.

"Mrs. Lempert, the bathtub is draining very slowly. I was standing in water six inches deep when I took my morning shower."

"I'll call the plumber today and see how fast we can take care of that, Mr. Hart."

"Mrs. Lempert, the freezer of my refrigerator doesn't keep my mousse firm. Please do something. I entertain a lot, and my chocolate mousse is a favorite dessert with my guests."

"You'll get the next new refrigerator that comes into the building even if I have to exchange it with someone else's. Will that be all right, Joseph?"

I figured that no one else would care that much about a mousse.

"Mrs. Lempert, there's water coming through the ceiling every time the person above me takes a shower."

"I'll go upstairs now and see if I can talk to Marylou about it. She's probably not closing her shower curtain all the way, and I'll get someone as quickly as I can to look at the floor around the bathtub, too."

"Mrs. Lempert, some idiot banged into my car on my way to work. The car is going to cost me a lot to fix. I'll need more time to get the rent to you."

"Well Angus, I'm glad you weren't hurt. Do you think you can give me a little bit each week until you catch up?"

Sometimes I approached a tenant. "Mr. Wright, I didn't receive a rent check from you, and it's the tenth of the month."

"Don't worry, Mrs. Lempert. The check is in the mail." Sometimes it was.

I used the same philosophy that my father had used for the store—keep the customer happy—only now it was keep the tenant happy—if possible. The building was fully occupied in a short time, but putting it in shape took months. Eventually it began to turn a profit. We put the money aside. I soon discovered his plans for the profit.

"I think it's time to look for another place. Can you go tomorrow with me?" my father asked.

"I don't know if I'll be able to take care of another place."

"You'll be able. How's two o'clock? I'll tell Marvin."

Once again we started a search, keeping to the Park Avenue section, and this time we found a seven-unit structure that I recognized immediately as a find. It had once been a stately mansion. With a sweeping staircase, curved windows, marble fireplaces, carved moldings, and many fine details, it still retained its charm. My father bought it. Prices were low, and he needed very little cash for a down payment.

I learned a great deal in a short time. There was no task too menial for me. I cleaned stoves, refrigerators, sinks, and toilets. I hauled garbage, shoveled paths for the postman when the snow fell, and I always carried a huge bunch of keys. I didn't even know about making a master key till later. Once we were doing well, I found some people to take over some of the heavy work, but I was still on call day and night should emergencies occur, and they did.

About eleven o'clock one night, I received a phone call from one of our tenants, a young lady. Whenever I saw her she looked voluptuous and sleepy-eyed. On this night her voice was tremulous.

"My boyfriend is afraid to leave the building to go home," she said.

"Why?" I envisioned flood or fire engulfing the surrounding area.

"His wife is waiting for him outside with a knife," she answered.

"I see." I frantically tried to think through the problem.

My first idea was to go to the scene of the drama and talk to the wife. This idea was vetoed by my family. I thought of calling the police, but I hesitated for fear of escalating the problem. I called our resident supervisor, a euphemism for the man who occasionally helped me when he felt like it. He agreed to go out to talk to the wife, and he actually calmed her down and took her home. The next day, I approached my tenant, who was "the other woman," in the love triangle.

"How is it you're going out with a married man?" I tried to be motherly and defend the institution of marriage at the same time.

"He promised to divorce his wife and marry me," she answered. "But it's been over a year, and he didn't tell her."

"I think you're wasting your time with this man." I went on about how she was too young and attractive to get herself into these no-win dangerous situations, but I suddenly realized she wasn't listening. *She really doesn't want to hear what I have to say,* I thought. I stopped talking and politely took my leave. A few months later I bumped into her on the stair, and she looked heavy. I thought she was gaining weight from frustration. Two weeks after that encounter, I was checking a plumbing problem in the building when I heard the wail of a baby. I traced it to her apartment and knocked on the door. She came out holding her infant. Of course, I cooed at the tiny baby and wished the mother and child well. Not long after that, she gave me notice and said she had found a larger place.

Almost always I was the one who showed the apartments when they became vacant. I chose the new tenants by my own system, a completely unprofessional way involving "gut feelings." At first I shied away from asking personal questions about salary, thinking it rude. I did ask a few questions about place of work, length of time at the job, and often I got the phone number of a character reference, undoubtedly the prospective tenant's best friend or relative. That we prospered illustrates the power of faith and determination or else unexplainable luck.

Infrequently, when I was not available to show an apartment, my father would take over. To my surprise, he could be less objective than I. He once rented an apartment to a young man who promised to pay the security deposit and the first month's rent after he moved in.

"How could you do this, Father? This guy has money troubles already, and who knows when or if he'll come through with the rent or security deposit?" I was exasperated.

"He said he needed a chance to get on his feet, and I remembered how hard it was for me when I didn't have no money," he explained. "I felt sorry for him."

The big difference between my father and Rocky, our new tenant, was that Rocky had no compulsion to meet his obligations. Soon his girlfriend moved in with him, and shortly after, a huge dog took up residence in the apartment. I had stipulated that we did not allow dogs, but they ignored all requests to remove the dog, who was half husky and half wolf. Frequently, I had to remind Rocky and his girlfriend, Griselda, that I was waiting for some kind of payment. Each time they said they needed more time to get on their feet.

"It would help if you both got jobs," I finally felt forced to say.

"We're living on bread and vinegar," Griselda snapped and looked at me with hostility.

"Why vinegar?" I asked, but by then they had slammed the door in my face.

I asked my teen-aged son, David, to go with me the next time I went there. Esther, my sister went with us, too. I had told them I was not pleased with the dog's expression. As we drew up to the building I asked them to wait outside for me, and if I did not come down in a few minutes to come to apartment six to look for me.

"Who's there?" Rocky called out, when I knocked on the apartment door.

"It's Mrs. Lempert."

Silence followed. Then I heard whispering and low growls. Suddenly the door was thrown open and the dog lunged at me, his forelegs reaching for my shoulders. I screamed with all the strength I had, and turned and ran.

"He won't hurt you," I heard Rocky call after me.

I flew out the front door. David and Esther were already standing there ready to storm the building.

"Let's just go," I gasped. "I don't want to go back up right now."

We piled into the car and drove away. I had no idea how to deal with such tenants, but not long after they crept away in the middle of the night, owing us money.

I did not remind my father his heart had clouded his judgment, nor did he rehash the errors I made. We had an unspoken agreement that, even if it was hard, we would do our best not to blame each other for mistakes. Instead we would try to learn from them. We muddled through those early years living through all kinds of misadventures, but we prospered.

CHAPTER TWENTY-FOUR

Garage Sales and Bikes

The bad news was that Lake Erie was dying, and so were the white fish in it. There was a time when the finest white fish lived in Lake Erie, and we received frequent shipments of them from Buffalo. They had come by truck, or often my Uncle Yitzrak would drive in to get his order and my father's, too. Now we were getting fewer shipments from Boston and Canada., as well. Because of pollution in so many bodies of water, fish was getting expensive. It was no longer a cheap meal. There were fewer customers buying fresh fish, and there was less fish to sell. By the sixties the Joseph Avenue customers who made gefilte fish and those who ate fish on Fridays had moved away. It was not the immigrant neighborhood of my childhood. The avenue had changed, and with it that whole section of the city.

My father moved from Hollenbeck Street because our big backyard, which almost took up a whole city block, abutted the store of a local supermarket chain, Star Supermarkets. The Star officials offered my father a small sum of money for the right of way through his backyard. The company wanted its trucks to enter from Clinton Avenue, which the supermarket faced, drive through our yard, and exit at Hollenbeck Street. My father felt that if big trucks came lumbering through his backyard to load or unload merchandise, the value of his house would decrease dramatically.

"Buy the whole property, with the house, or don't buy nothing," he told the negotiator. The house and land were sold to Star Supermarkets in 1962. My father bought another double house not far from Dan and me on Harvard Street. He lived on one side and rented the other side. I, of course, handled the renting.

It was a big change for my father, moving to another part of town. He could no longer walk to his synagogue on the Sabbath or holidays. He had been a charter member of B'nai Israel, his sole place of worship for over thirty years. He continued for a while to go there during the week, but he also joined a synagogue within walking distance of Harvard Street, Beth Sholom. There he went on the Sabbath and all the holidays. Eventually he went there for every prayer service.

In the late Friday afternoon of July 24, 1964, my father closed early enough to prepare for the Sabbath. As usual, the whole family gathered at his house, bringing our prearranged contributions to the Sabbath dinner. I enjoyed our times together. Esther was in top form. She had recently finished a theatrical run of a play in which she had a significant role. Her descriptions of the misadventures behind the scenes were hilarious. She was unsurpassed as a mimic and raconteur. She picked up facial expressions and nuances of voice. We were breathless with laughter. None of us knew that within hours a violent uprising bringing destruction would crash down, engulf Joseph Avenue, and change it forever. The race riots started that night.

We did not know that thousands of people were rioting in the streets. In the ensuing chaos people smashed store windows, throwing bricks and rocks. They vandalized the stores, emptying them of merchandise. Fires were started. When the police chief went down to survey the scene, his car was overturned. In the middle of the night the city manager declared a state of emergency. The state troopers were called in at 3 A.M. They, along with the city police and sheriff's deputies, could not quell the rioting from spreading to the Third Ward. I didn't know what was happening until a friend called me Saturday morning to find out if we knew whether the store had sustained much damage.

Saturday morning my father went to Sabbath services as he always did. He would not drive to Joseph Avenue on the Sabbath to assess the damage. Even if he had wanted to, he couldn't have gone because the police had set up a twenty-block perimeter to contain the rioting. By Sunday night, the National Guard had been called in. When I saw pictures of people on Joseph Avenue beset by the police with dogs on the front page of the New York Times, I felt a stab of deep pain. The avenue which I remembered as a street of hope and vitality was now littered and devastated, the embodiment of despair and hopelessness.

When we finally got to our store the next day we saw that it had not been touched. My father was relieved and happy. "You see," he declared, "my neighbors like me. They know I treat everyone the same."

"Father, what's happening is bigger than just having your neighbors like you. I think the rioting didn't spread as far as Clifford Avenue. Most of the trouble stopped a block or two away from the store." He thought I was wrong, and his store was untouched by design.

After the riot, many businesses left the area. My father saw no reason to move away. He liked his neighborhood, and he liked his customers, whoever they were and as few as they might be. With less fish to sell and fewer customers, my father did make some concessions. He began going to work later in the day. There was no need to get up at dawn to chop ice, and ready all the boxes of fish. He no longer rolled the big barrels of herring or pickles or black olives outside to line them up at the store front. Indeed, who would have bought the schmaltz herring or olives or dill pickles? A new generation of shoppers did not want to come down to Joseph Avenue to shop. Many younger housewives bought their herring and pickles and olives in jars from the supermarket. They bought their gefilte fish in jars.

Most men my father's age retired and enjoyed their leisure, relaxing or taking up hobbies. We daughters encouraged our father to retire, but he brushed such suggestions aside. He was in his mid-sixties and still strong and full of energy. He may have spent fewer hours in the store, but he still enjoyed going there and talking to customers, both old and new.

"I open the store when I want to. I close up when I want to," he said. "I'm not working hard."

It must have been about this time that my father's enjoyment of buying and selling found an outlet in garage sales. He discovered all kinds of bargains that he brought to the store to sell. His shelves slowly began to fill up with dishes, wearing apparel, appliances, knickknacks and an odd assortment of merchandise. The customers responded positively to his new line of goods by buying much of what he put up for sale. He had developed his own method of searching out bargains. Early on Sunday he surveyed the garage sale scene, and if the price was right, he made his purchases. If the prices were not right, he returned at the end of the day and bought the items he wanted, most often reduced in price by then. His strategy was to come by just as the last browsers of the day were leaving a garage sale. The garage salesperson might have begun to tiredly pack up his leftovers—the articles that had not sold.

"How much do you want for all the stuff on this table?" my father told me he asked. Sometimes a little negotiating was required, but a deal was usually struck, with both sides pleased. My father would scoop up his bargains and take them all to the store. He had room to tastefully display his garage sale wares because there were fewer boxes of fish and fewer grocery items. In front of the remaining fish boxes where raw fish stared in amazed surprise, he had lined up shoes— men's, women's children's. Some were a little run down, but others were in fairly good shape.

A housewife might come in for some Campbell's tomato soup and leave with a pair of leather gloves, a little frayed at the finger tips but still quite wearable. Perhaps a young matron would ask for five pounds of sugar and my father would take the opportunity to show her a set of drinking glasses.

"I'm selling it cheap, Missus, because one is missing and one is chipped a little bit. You can't hardly see where."

To another he advised, "I think you need a new sweater. What you're wearing is looking very bad." She had come in to buy a can of peas, and he held up a sweater to interest her.

"Do you need a toaster?" he might question a housewife. "This one works very good."

A slight, somewhat shabby-looking older man came in one time and asked my father if he had any pants to sell. My father, undoubtedly using long dormant skills from his days in the clothing industry, assured his customer that he could outfit him perfectly. Rummaging through a pile of neatly folded pants that he had next to the display of Maxwell House Coffee, my father pulled out a navy-blue pair. Holding it up and measuring his customer with his eyes, my father suggested the man try it on over his old pants to see if it would fit. I watched fascinated, as this transaction evolved. The pants, even over the customer's clothes, were a little loose, but he seemed pleased.

"Here's a belt. I'll throw it in for nothing," my father said. "You already look better from when you came in."

Customers began bringing him articles they hoped to sell. Some of them might not have had very much cash and wanted to barter. He might accept a pair of men's work pants or a few pairs of socks, if they met his not too exacting standards, in exchange for a fish or grocery order. By the late sixties the store began to resemble a second hand store or thrift shop. The special of the week was prominently displayed in the store front window. The special was always a bicycle.

My son, David, who was then thirteen, was building bikes in our garage and bringing them to my father to sell. David had listened to his own father tell of how he had put together his first bicycle from bits and pieces of old bicycle parts. Dan had often reminisced about the Great Depression and had told David that, "In my day" he had had to figure out how to make what they could not afford to buy.

David began to spend many hours trying to put together a bicycle from the parts he found in the trash that people left in front of their house for the garbage collectors. He rode around the neighborhood and beyond, looking for discarded bicycles. If he could not get these bicycle skeletons to our house alone, he enlisted our help. We drove over and picked them up in our car and deposited them in our garage. Several times he found a pile of bicycle frames near the railroad tracks where he walked to East High School (which was also a junior high at that time). He wondered why there were so many frames there. He brought home whatever he found. Suddenly there were no bike frames left near

145

the tracks. Their appearance and disappearance remained a mystery, although someone suggested long afterward that those bike frames might have come from stolen bicycles.

David saved all the parts he found and had a large inventory of parts from which to choose. At one point he had several big boxes of parts and twenty complete bikes. With every bike he made, he grew more expert. Occasionally neighborhood children came to our house to buy a bike.

Like all the grandchildren, he had worked in his grandfather's store on Sundays from the time he was eight or nine. All of them, boys and girls alike, spent some time in the store learning a little philosophy and salesmanship from my father.

He told them all, "You got to give the customers what they want—good, cheap merchandise, good service." He taught his young helpers to say, "Thank you, call again," at the end of every transaction. David wanted to say, "Thanks a lot," but my father demanded that everyone say it his way: "Thank you, call again." Nobody argued with Grandfather.

David loved unpacking cartons of groceries and displaying them in an attractive arrangement. Instead of piling cans on top of each other, he believed his triangular groupings of cans added interest to the merchandise displays in the store. All the children dusted cans, cleaned the display cooler, swept the floor, and sometimes waited on customers. Gail's favorite job was sitting behind the cash register, making change. She still remembered, years later, that at the end of her "shift" a can of Purple Passion pop was her reward. Alan recalled weighing out one-pound bags of dried split peas from a fifty-pound bag. That was one of the most tiresome tasks, but Alan didn't complain. Jeff, who later became a business man himself, busied himself dusting the displays. Paul, Maureen, and Randy also served their apprenticeship. Judy recalls that her grandfather held her up so she could press the cash register keys. In a year or more most of them became too busy or found other interests, and they no longer had time to go to the store.

David, however, now had a lucrative business partnership with his grandfather. He searched for old bicycles, repaired or remade them, and gave them to his grandfather to sell. Whatever the bicycle could be sold for was turned over to David. My father took no commission.

My son said he never forgot the lessons he learned from his Grampa. One of my father's axioms was, "You gotto spend money to make money." David learned to buy a needed part if the part would make the bike work better.

"It didn't take me too long to figure out that if I spent the money to buy a necessary part, the finished bike would bring more than enough money to pay for the part and still make a profit.

"Grampa wanted me to find out what a secondhand bike was worth, and what we could sell it for. He told me his customers could not pay a lot. I learned to cover my costs and then ask for a little more. The bikes in the window never stayed there more than a week."

Once when David delivered a bicycle to the store and it didn't sell fast, my father brought it back to him. He told David that it wasn't selling because the wheels were rusty.

"You need to clean them," his grandfather said. He made David understand that seeing rusty wheels turned people off. It didn't look good, and maybe people felt there were other things wrong.

"If you want to sell your bicycles for the right price you have to do everything you can to improve them," my father told him. This advice annoyed David at first. He wanted to sell his bikes as quickly as possible, but he knew his grandfather dealt directly with the customer. He respected his grandfather's experience and wisdom.

"I learned to 'detail' the bikes," David told me much later. He came to appreciate how important it was to pay attention to details. He was becoming a craftsman.

So, as David spent Sundays working on bikes, my father spent Sundays driving around looking for garage sales. Business was booming, and their partnership was thriving. On the morning of July 9th, 1972, everything stopped.

CHAPTER TWENTY-FIVE

After the Attack

He was on his way to Sunday morning services when he decided to stop at the store. A "tall, good-looking man" came in and asked for money. Although my father gave him what he had, the robber strangled him into unconsciousness and gouged out his eyes.

I was the last person he saw, because he stopped by our house to pick up his car Saturday night after the Sabbath. When he moved to Harvard Street, only a block away from Dan and me, it was easy for him to park his car in one of our garages on Friday before sundown and pick it up Saturday night after sundown. That Saturday night in July, he came in to talk a little bit, as he usually did, before driving his old Chevy out. We chatted briefly, and as he left he said, "I'll see you tomorrow."

I nodded, called out after him, "Okay," and returned to the book I had been reading.

He never saw me again. Could I have changed the course of events by doing or saying something that night? If I had talked to him longer, kept him in my house for an hour or two would he have been tired enough to sleep a little later the next morning, open the store even 20 minutes later? I thought, too, of the offhand way I had let him go out. Why didn't I walk him to the door, maybe give him a quick kiss in farewell, really look at him?

My father never saw my sisters and me again. He never saw us grow older. He did not see his grandchildren mature into adults, but he heard them, he talked to them, and he listened to them. He felt the small hands of the children grow larger as each child grew up. He put his hand out to greet them when they came to see him. Paul began shaking my father's hand and putting a cellophane-wrapped piece of hard candy in it. Often Paul said nothing when he came in, but the minute my father felt the piece of candy, he smiled and said, "Pauli."

When I visited my father I usually took his right hand and held it for a moment, telling him, "It's Ruth, Father."

He then put his thumb and middle finger around my wrist and always said to me, "You're too thin. Are you eating enough?" Invariably, I laughed and assured him I was.

My father loved having visits from all of us. He enjoyed being with the family. He argued and laughed, and discussed weighty matters with each one. He never stopped trying to have his own way which in itself initiated more arguments and discussions.

His blindness did not diminish his influence on the family—it served, rather, to intensify it. He was the center of our holiday celebrations and our family gatherings. Thrust upon him at the age of seventy-two, his blindness did not shove him into the background of our lives. Instead it pulled us together even more as we all rearranged our lives again. I wondered how he managed to exert such influence on us. What was the source of his power over all his family from the youngest grandchild to the oldest of his daughters? Despite his blindness, each and every one of us went to great lengths to help him live the kind of life he wanted to live.

Our commitment to preserving for him the life he knew had actually begun years earlier when my mother died. We learned then to pull together, but I knew, as people outside the family did not know, that although we all pulled together, not everyone wanted to pull the same way. There were differences in temperament, different priorities—of career, of social aspirations, of education. The challenge was to handle the differences effectively and with grace. Now that we had more interaction than even before, I had to learn to keep my mouth shut. I had argued with a couple of my brothers-in-law quite regularly, sometimes descending to yells and name calling.

One Saturday afternoon, as the family sat together after our Sabbath lunch, we were discussing women's rights, a new and popular topic of discussion then. The conversation had gone quite well, when it suddenly took an unfortunate turn. Voices were rising, someone's hand pounded the table. Before I knew it I was shouting, "You're a male chauvinist pig," to my opinionated brother-in-law.

One of my sisters ran over to my adversary and whispered in his ear, "You know what Ruth's like. Stop arguing with her."

Another sister grabbed my arm and said, "Stop yelling, and quit taking everything so seriously." We both backed down and apologized to each other.

I discovered that trying to win an argument or having the last word all the time did not make me feel good. I loved my sisters more than I liked winning an argument with their husbands. Despite that love, there were conflicts among us, times of hurt feelings, moments of jealousy and anger. We learned to make concessions, but I came to slowly realize we could better enjoy our times together if we overlooked or forgave each other our failings—or at least appeared to. Our father exemplified for us the strength and courage of family. He suffused us with his sense of belonging and kinship. With his example in mind we believed that together we could overcome whatever difficulties there might be.

Every holiday and every Sabbath meal meant there might be as many as fourteen or more sitting down at the table, possibly fewer if someone had other commitments. Our arrangements were relatively loose. As the children became teenagers they were not always there, but they knew they were welcome whenever they came. They were encouraged to drop by to say hello even if they couldn't stay.

Our children had been young when my mother died, and we first began our Sabbath arrangements. Like the postman, my sisters and our families had slogged through snow and ice, sleet and rain, heat and sunshine, to get to my father's house every Friday and Saturday with freshly made chicken soup and noodles, roast brisket with potatoes or maybe rice, salad and dessert. In the winter when the sun set early we raced wildly to get to his house before he came home so we could start reheating the meal. We could not turn the stove on during the Sabbath because that was against religious practice. I laughingly offered to be the "Shabbos goy," but he laughingly, but firmly refused that request.

Because the children were babies, we came with all our paraphernalia—diaper bags, play pens, toys, and extra outfits. The place looked like a nursery. When the grandchildren were old enough, my father walked with them—sometimes all eight—to Cobbs Hill Park on Saturday afternoon after our midday Sabbath meal. My sisters and I rushed in various directions to catch up on errands. The children loved their time with Grandpa at Cobb's Hill. He always treated them to candy or ice cream from the concession stand. The children noticed that money did not change hands.

"How come we can get an ice cream cone or a candy bar without paying for them?" Paul asked. The children believed that because he was religious and observant, he had special powers that the concession owner recognized. He did not tell them he had paid ahead of time so he would not have to handle money on Saturday. On the way to their excursion to the park they all stopped at the cannon in front of the armory on Culver Road. Showing off his strength, my father shook the cannon. The children never forgot how strong he was and were impressed. They always came running to us afterward to tell us of this feat of strength.

His imperious demands on our time did not diminish our regard. We greeted his suggestion of a family trip to Israel with enthusiasm. Our plans were in high gear. The excitement kept rising. And then the brutal attack, like a steel beam thrown in front of a speeding train, derailed us. Our careful plans lay broken. Our belief in the future shattered. We looked at each other in the hospital as he lay in the emergency room. How could this be? What should we do? It was my father who pointed the way.

By his willingness to go on the trip to Israel a month after being attacked, he signaled to us that he was not going to let his blindness interfere with his plans. When he began taking every course available to him we saw that he planned to keep and sustain his interest in the world around him—that he had no time for bitterness or self-pity. His insistence that we all participate in holiday celebrations while he spearheaded the plans, assured us that he did not expect to languish on the sidelines. His moments of grief he kept mainly to himself. I told him once that many of my friends thought he was brave, and that they were inspired by his positive outlook. He said, "How would you feel if I sat all day and complained? Wouldn't the whole family feel bad if I cried all the time? It would make things worse. What would I accomplish?" He was following the advice he had given each of us—you have to keep moving,

Even when it's hard. Even when it seems impossible.

CHAPTER TWENTY-SIX

Grandchildren

Because my three sisters and I were together every week, the children played together while we prepared the meals in my father's house. With Alan, the oldest, as the ringleader, they appropriated one of the upstairs bedrooms. As we set the table we heard them cavorting overhead. The sound of laughter, thumps, bumps, and sometimes crashes assailed our ears. We admonished them to be careful, sometimes going up to assess the damage. Their grandfather was not particularly concerned with their uninhibited playing, but he was a little testy when they broke a chair. Those children, some now in middle age, remember with surprising clarity all those Fridays and Saturdays.

As they grew older the grandchildren went to him for advice. They asked his opinion on matters of business and sometimes, matters of the heart. With Paul, his grandson who went into business for himself, he discussed cash flow and effective advertising. To another he might point out the problems of intermarriage as he saw it. He had a good time dancing at his grandchildren's weddings. He loved a party, and he enjoyed every celebration. He flew to Israel with Esther and Jerry to attend the wedding of granddaughter, Maureen. When that marriage fell apart he was saddened, but his love and support did not waver.

Harriet's house was our base of operations for holiday celebrations, but all of us shopped and cooked for every single holiday, because he celebrated them all. I thought we had more meetings to arrange our Passover seders than a five-star general planning a campaign. One of the more difficult problems involved setting up the temporary dwelling, the "Sukkey," for the holiday of Sukkoth. The "Sukkey" was a four-sided abode with slats across the top that served as a roof. Whoever was inside could look up and see the sky and the stars. The holiday came in late fall, so there was usually rain and cold to contend with as we sat and ate in the "Sukkey." My father felt it incumbent for everyone to eat in this small replica of what the ancient Hebrews might have used and to suffer whatever vicissitudes they might have suffered, such as eating with the wind and rain sweeping over us.

The problem was that the "Sukkey" had to be put together within a brief time. The boys and the men of the family often grumbled because they felt there was so little time to construct it, and to hang the apples and grapes from the slats. Everyone complained, but almost everyone pitched in, and we always finished just in time.

Each of the grandchildren had special memories of him. Judy told us that he came over to coach her as she prepared for her Bat Torah. Alan went to him to co-sign a loan when he bought his first car. Randy felt that he could hear his grandfather's voice advising him in some moments of uncertainty or difficulty. Gail recalls many of his favorite sayings and made a list of them. Some of his favorites:

"Let's keep moving," when he was dissatisfied with the rate of speed of anything that was happening, or when he wanted to move forward.

"One false move and it's good-bye, Charlie," used to describe some of the dangerous or tricky situations he found himself in.

"This is a job for a policeman," when a job or task seemed overwhelming.

"Believe everybody, but don't trust nobody," a reminder to all of us not to be too gullible.

"We want action," said to anyone who was sitting around apparently not doing something useful, also used as a substitute for, *"Let's keep moving."*

He also had singular pronunciations of words he used often, such as "oombelievable" (unbelievable) used to express wonderment or, in some cases, dismay. At a gathering to celebrate an anniversary he would happily say, "Happy University."

Jeffry looked back at the times he spent dusting all the cans and displays. He tried to be meticulous even though it was a tiresome task.

Paul started smoking at a young age and became a heavy smoker. One Sunday afternoon he was watching a football game, drinking beer and smoking, when he received a call from his grandfather, who asked him what he was doing. Paul said he was watching TV, relaxing, and smoking.

"Isn't it time you stopped smoking?"

Paul thought about it for a few minutes and decided to stop immediately. "I quit cold turkey," he said.

Such was my father's influence.

Maureen never wanted to disappoint him. If she was admonished for a wrongdoing she asked her mother not to tell Grandpa. When the county legislature asked for nominations for family of the year in 1983, Maureen wrote a letter nominating our family with, her grandfather as its patriarch. Four families were chosen for the honor. Maureen won for our family. She accompanied my father to the award ceremony. It was a proud and happy time for us all.

CHAPTER TWENTY-SEVEN

Second Journey

He kept learning new skills, gaining confidence, testing his ability to be independent. Before long he began talking about traveling again. Believing as he did in the power of education, and feeling that travel is a major component of education, my father suggested that we plan a second family trip. I checked school schedules, work plans, and vacation dates. Harriet, Esther, and I consulted a travel agent. Marcia and her family did not choose to go. Of our subsequent trips, Howard went on one other. Marcia went on most of the trips alone.

With our agent the three of us looked through tour books, trip brochures, and itineraries, unable to find a trip that would suit our financial and special needs. My father would not travel on the Sabbath during a trip. Finally our agent pulled out a trip brochure. "This might be just right for your father and the rest of you, too," she said. "It's called "Jewish Highlights of Europe." She described a two-week trip sponsored by the Israeli Airlines that included three capitals of Europe—London, Madrid, and Paris. I looked at the itinerary, noticing that on weekends there were no planned activities or change of place requiring travel. There was ample free time for our individual sightseeing.

Deciding I needed to begin practicing my rusty French immediately, I shouted, "Voila!" which I translated to mean, "We have found our trip."

The rest were just as enthusiastic. It was a smaller group of us that departed in mid-August. Along with my father were the Seigels, the Usdanes, and the Lemperts. The evening of August 16, 1973, was almost a year to the day of our first trip. We sat at LaGuardia in the El Al terminal that night, eager to begin our second travel adventure together. Although we were to take seven family trips, we never lost this excitement for our travels. I was full of wonder and surprise that we, unsophisticated and unworldly, were actually going to see more of the world again.

"Let's keep moving. Why are we all still sitting around?" my father asked.

"Father, we're still waiting for the plane to arrive. I'm sure it won't be long before we'll be boarding," Esther assured him. Sure enough, we were soon airborne.

Naomi, the guide who met our tired group at Heathrow Airport at ten the next morning, guided us to the Imperial Hotel. Although most of us had been unable to sleep on the plane, we were too excited to rest. We sat down with Naomi in the lobby of the Imperial and listened as she made suggestions for restaurants, places of worship, and explained our options for sightseeing. She was prepared to help us make arrangements for excursions and a possible evening at the theater. Because it was Friday, I explained that my father expected us to find a place of worship, if not for that night, then for Saturday. She told us where we could find a kosher meal and gave us the address of a synagogue not too far from our hotel.

While my father rested and the others walked about and breathed in the British air, Dan and I found our way to Hillel House to make reservations for the Sabbath noon meal, which my father would enjoy after Saturday morning services. With the reservations completed for those of us who would go to Sabbath services and lunch, we went back to the hotel and told everyone we were ready to begin our usual routine, involving my father. First, we discovered which of our rooms was the "best" one for him. David and my father exchanged rooms with Esther and Jerry. We could then begin our orientation for my father. Harriet deftly moved a few pieces of furniture to expedite matters. He practiced moving around the room under our supervision until we were all satisfied that he could manage to find his way without trouble. That night we all went to a nearby restaurant for dinner. My father pronounced the fish excellent. We went back to the hotel with him well before sundown.

Saturday morning several of us got up early, dressed carefully, and knocked at my father's door. He was ready and waiting. Harriet always laid out his clothes the night before. He could then dress without assistance in the morning. It took us 45 minutes to walk to the Dean Street Synagogue, which was unexpectedly closed.

"What's the matter with them? I never heard of closing up shul on Shabbos," my father said, annoyed. We assured him we would find another one. On our map we found the Hallam Street Synagogue, and after another 45 minute walk we arrived. My father was a fast walker, but we managed to keep up with him.

I was surprised to see that the president of the shul and the rabbi wore top hats, a customary practice in England. Except for that, the chants and the Hebrew prayers were the same that we would have been hearing and reading back home. The same portion of the Torah was being read in every synagogue in the world. We talked and chatted with the English worshippers after services, but excused ourselves to walk to Hillel House where our Sabbath meal awaited us. My father enjoyed his chicken soup immensely. We met a number of young people there, one of whom was Ayoub, whose family sold Persian rugs. He wanted us to visit his family's warehouse.

"We have all sizes of carpets. I will see that you get a very good bargain. Here is my card," he said, handing it to me. In the next few days I tried to find someone to go to the warehouse with me, but no one wanted to see Persian rugs. Everyone was too busy sightseeing.

On Sunday a little bus picked us up and took us through the old city of London. Our guide led us through the ghetto where the Jews had lived. We saw an old Sephardic synagogue dating from 1701, although the congregation itself was even older than the building. We looked with admiration at the Marble Arch Synagogue, fairly new and impressive. In the Jewish Museum we described to my father the beautiful mezuzahs, intricately designed ketubahs, and the old relics on display.

Returning to our hotel to freshen up, all of us were ready for more exploring on our own. With my father exhorting us to keep moving we found our way to the Tower of London, and there we took turns telling my father about Ann Boleyn.

"They took off her head right here," Paul told him. My father shook his own head in dismay. In the days that followed we saw the changing of the guard at Buckingham Palace, walked through Trafalgar Square, gazed in awe at Westminster Abbey, marveled a the food displays in Harrods. When Harriet described to my father the dazzling array of food, my father shook his head, this time in wonderment.

We visited the British Museum. Here, one of the guards broke the "DO NOT TOUCH" rule and guided my father's hand over the sculptures. My father listened as we explained the Rosetta Stone, The Elgin Marbles, the Egyptian monuments. The next day, with my father urging us not to waste a minute, we visited Windsor Castle, Hampton Palace, and Waddeston Manor, Baron Rothschild's home.

We all wanted to see a play, and Naomi assured us she had found the perfect play, one that would be suitable for the age range of our group. As I sat in the darkened theater and watched *Grease,* I was extremely uncomfortable that my father and our young offspring were exposed to the profanity and situations depicted in the play.

Calling Harriet and Esther together after the show, I said, "Isn't it ironic that we saw an American play here in London that I would never have taken our kids to see back home? I think its message is completely unsuitable for the children. I'm going to make sure it doesn't happen again." Then and there I appointed myself the watchdog of morality for any future entertainment that we would plan as a group. Esther and Harriet did not disagree, sensing, no doubt, that I was firm in my resolve.

After four exciting days in London we were on the plane heading for Spain. How warm and welcome were the heat and the bright sunlight. One of the highlights of Madrid was a flamenco show that all of us enjoyed except for the two youngest—Gail now 12 and Randy almost

10. We all wanted them to go with us, but by law they were not permitted because wine was served during the show.

"Won't you all come to my home?" our tour guide, Carmen, asked when the entertainment was over

"Si, Si," I replied for all of us. I was the most proficient in Spanish.

Carmen lived in a large, gracious apartment that had once seen better days. I noticed cobwebs in the corners and on the high ceiling. We observed cracked plaster and peeling paint on the walls. Her family had once been very wealthy, she told us.

"We lose everything in the war," she explained, meaning the Spanish Civil War. Her father had been a high-ranking official before the war. She had been five or six when the war started. She remembered her father's execution. She recalled how her family had suffered a complete reversal of fortune.

"Tonight I open a special bottle of wine for you in honor of your father," she said. "I have saved it for a long time, and now I want you all to have some."

"Here, let me help you open that bottle," Jerry offered, and began wrestling with the cork.

After a brief struggle he uncorked the wine and she poured a little into several glasses. We were enjoying her hospitality, but I thought that she carried within her a sadness that never seemed to lift. Even when she laughed or smiled, her eyes were somber. Paul made a toast to Carmen and everyone drank to her. I had asked for water, citing an intolerance to alcohol, but I noticed some strange expressions as the drinkers took their first sip. We all kept chatting amiably, but one by one, someone left the room, glass in hand, and returned with an empty glass. When we made our farewells Carmen pressed a lovely piece of Lladro sculpture into my father's hand, and insisted he take it home. All of us thanked her for so delightful an evening.

"I don't know how long she had that wine but something was sure wrong with it. It must have turned," Jerry remarked as we walked to the corner of the street looking for taxis. We all poured our wine into a plant. "Maybe it'll grow better." I was glad that Carmen did not know about it.

The next afternoon we visited the Prado, once again describing to my father many of the masterpieces—telling him of their artistry as we saw it, their religious significance, their overwhelming size. "Father, the picture we're looking at is the size of the living room wall in your house."

He, wearing his skullcap, shook his head from side to side, again in wonderment. "Oombelievable," he said.

Shopping in Madrid was a favorite pastime for the shoppers in our group. During the daily siesta time, shops, stores, and restaurants were closed. The shoppers had to arrange their schedule to shop later in the day or evening. One day we all elected to take a bus ride to Toledo. We walked down the narrow, sun-baked streets, stopping to visit El Greco's house, then to tour an ancient synagogue. On a free afternoon everyone went swimming in the pool on the hotel's roof. My father loved splashing in the cool water, and we all found it refreshing.

After four days in Madrid we were on our way to Orly Airport in Paris.

CHAPTER TWENTY-EIGHT

Another Success

Paris was full of culinary and cultural delight. Cynthia, our tour guide in Paris, spoke English without any trace of an accent. I marveled at her fluency. "Where did you learn to speak English like an American?" I asked

"Brooklyn," she replied. "That's where I was born." Cynthia was young, attractive, and chic. She made suggestions on places to see and things to do.

"We'd like to see a French show that would be suitable for the whole family," I said, emphasizing the ages of the young people and the word "suitable." She recommended a revue playing at the Casino de Paris. "It has music, magicians, acrobats, and dancers."

"It sounds perfect," said Esther.

"Just the thing for all of us," added Harriet. Judy and David, my teenagers, thought it would be fun. Maureen and Paul, also in their teens, agreed, and so did Gail and Randy, the youngest. I was probably more excited than they were.

When we arrived at the theater and were taken to our seats I was pleased to notice that we were advancing to the very front of the theater.

"We're so close to the front that we'll feel as though we're sitting on the stage," I joked.

"We are sitting on the stage," Harriet answered as we climbed the few steps up to the stage. We were very much to the side so that it was difficult to get the full view of the stage. Our seats did not obscure the view of anyone in the audience. The performers, however, had to practically step over us when they made their exits and entrances.

Not long after we were ensconced in our seats the band struck up a lively tune, and out onto the stage leapt a dozen or so voluptuous young women, topless and otherwise scantily clad. We all gazed in astonishment at the bouncing breasts, wiggling hips and high-kicking thighs and legs. True, there were magicians and acrobats, but the dancing girls were most memorable. My youngest sister, Harriet, saw that the comely performers were brushing by Randy so closely that the feathers they wore as costumes were tickling Randy at every entrance and exit. Not only that, their ample bosoms were almost hitting Randy in the face. Harriet turned to Dan and asked, "Won't you please change places with Randy?"

"Of course, of course," he replied, too eager to oblige, I thought. He did not mind being tickled at all. The teenagers seemed to be enthralled by the show.

"Is everyone having a good time?" my father turned to me and asked. "I could truthfully tell him that the costumes, music, and dancing were spectacular, and that all eyes were glued to the stage.

One evening Esther asked, "How about going to a French night club that the chamber maid said was very good?" Our maid spoke very little English, and Esther knew no French, so it was a mystery to me how she could get into a conversation about nightclubs, but I trusted Esther to find good places to have a good time. No one knew how to find, make, or enjoy a party better than Esther. When it came to having fun I would gladly follow her suggestions anywhere, anytime.

Harriet and Bob stayed with their children. Esther, Jerry, Dan, and I took the Metro to the Michou, a small intimate club with a red-lacquered ceiling and walls of glittering silver that lent an atmosphere of excitement and drama. At a little round table the four of us sat sipping French wine, feeling worldly as we looked at the other patrons and smiling at the good-looking waiters who were so attentive and friendly. "Isn't that beautiful girl at the next table wearing Chanel No. 5?" Esther leaned over and said to me. "I'm going to look for some tomorrow."

"Maybe it costs less here," I answered.

"Why does that waiter keep looking at me?" Dan whispered. "He's come over twice to ask me if he can get me something."

"He's probably looking at me, Dan. He thinks we're rich Americans and big tippers, so he keeps coming over to our table. He's in for a big disappointment on both counts." When the waiter handed me the menu, I knew it would be challenging, but I recognized coq au vin and quickly ordered it. It was one of the best dinners I ever ate.

With a roll of drums the show started, and we were all enthralled by the lilting music and the beautiful chorus line of shapely singers and dancers. The performers wore dazzling gowns, tight and sparkling with sequins and beads. All of them had beautiful hair, intricately and elaborately arranged. They sang rather daring songs, and moved in a seductive way

"They are all so gorgeous, so seductive, and so truly womanly," I said to Esther. "I can always spot a French woman. She has more oomph than the rest of us."

It seemed to me the show was over too soon. I kept clapping, hoping we might get an encore or two. The performers kept bowing and blowing kisses in all directions. Suddenly all of them put their hands to their head and pulled off their hair, disclosing closely cropped heads, and thick muscular necks.

"They're all men?" I said in amazement

Jerry who was apparently the most observant of us said, "I think we're among the few straight people here." I looked at the waiter who was coming back to our table.

Yes, I thought, *he really is looking at Dan.*

Wherever we went we took public transportation as much as possible, because the subway system in London and Paris could quickly take us anywhere. However, a long and steep escalator was the only way we could reach the Tube or the Metro. I had taken my father on the escalator once, and both of us nearly toppled down the huge moving stairs. My brothers-in-law soon devised a method that eliminated all risk. Every time we went down or came up from the subway my father had a son-in-law on each arm. They would sing in unison, "One, two, three," and all three men would step on the escalator at the same time with my father held firmly in the middle.

We took the metro to the Louvre. The doorman refused to charge my father an admission fee. We all split up, and I took my father to "see" the Mona Lisa, and the Venus de Milo. We walked slowly along so I could explain some of the paintings to him. Before long Harriet took his arm and guided him to some of her favorites, as I ran to find the Winged Victory, a sculpture that I had wanted to view since taking an art-history course in college many years before. When I found the Winged Victory on the stair, I stood before her, feeling the wind that swirled around her garment.

That night we took the Seine River boat ride with Paris illuminated. "Father, we're gliding down the river in the middle of Paris," Harriet told him. Each of the children went to his side to describe the shimmering lights, the night sky, the reflections on the water, and the city gleaming around us. The next afternoon we went to the Eiffel Tower, taking a cage up to the second level where my father bought his favorite dessert, ice cream.

One day we went on a Jewish Past and Present tour, viewing the Pletzel, the old Jewish section of Paris with its tiny synagogue. We bought a challah at a little kosher bakery. It was later at the Palace of Versailles that I became ill—light headed and faint.

"You have a slight green tinge to your face," said Harriet, always the nurse. The security guard, afraid that I might become sick on the carpeting, rushed me down to the basement. Harriet left the others to accompany me and Dan; the three of us missed the garden tour. I felt better sitting in the cool dankness of the basement than in the sunny brightness above.

"I'm sorry you're missing the end of the palace tour," I told Harriet.

She dismissed my apology, and said, "No one else is seeing the dungeons and underground passages that we're seeing."

Although I felt better the next day, I rested. There was so much more I had wanted to see. It was our last day, and the others tried to spend their time absorbing more of Paris. That evening I told my father I could not leave Paris without walking down the Champs Elysees. "Will you go with me?" I asked. "I'm feeling better."

"Let's get moving," he said, grabbing his guide stick.

We picked up a few other family members eager to join us, took the Metro, and within minutes we were walking down The Champs Elysees. The air was soft, the night was warm, and it was thrilling to be strolling along that majestic boulevard.

"Father, the stores are so elegant," I told him. "There's a beautiful shop with gorgeous clothes in the window."

"Now we're passing a leather store," Esther told him. "The handbags are elegant."

"They must cost a fortune," my father remarked, ever the practical merchant.

On the plane homeward the next day, I felt a momentary twinge of regret for all that I had not seen. Quickly I looked around me and saw the faces of the family talking and laughing, someone always walking down the aisle to see my father. None of us could do exactly as we wanted. The splendor of the trip and every trip we were to take, was not only in what we saw and did and learned. It was that we were creating memories of our family together—for ourselves and for our children.

CHAPTER TWENTY-NINE

Shopping

Once home we went back to our routines. One of my father's favorite pastimes was shopping. He enjoyed buying as much as selling. I remembered his telling me that when he was a child in Poland he bought eggs and dairy products from their land owner as well as items from the villagers and sold them all in the market in the next town. He also bought some foods in the market and sold them in his village. Did he enjoy it so much that he decided to become a storekeeper when he came to the New World? Is the love of the marketplace something you inherit? He was such a natural salesman, I wondered if he had learned from his parents the art of selling and buying or if it was in his blood.

After he was blinded and the store was closed, he still wanted to go shopping with me. He and I would buy most of what we needed for our weekly Friday night family dinners. He preferred the public market to the super market, so that was often where we shopped.

"We need potatoes," he said one cold winter morning. "Let's go to the market." I had just come into Harriet's house and was taking off my coat.

"Father, it's too cold to go to the public market. That place is twenty degrees colder than any place else on earth. You'll freeze," I admonished him.

"Don't worry about me. We need potatoes, so let's get moving." He touched his talking clock to get the time.

"It's late. What took you so long today?" he questioned.

Dismissing further argument, he put on his coat, gloves, and fake-fur hat. Seeing that he was determined, I handed him his muffler, made sure he had his guide stick, put my coat back on, and we sallied forth into the wintry morning.

The public market was relatively quiet on Thursdays compared to Saturdays. Absent were the crush of people, the jumble of a myriad of voices and languages, the hawking of foodstuffs by the vendors, the loud voices of people calling to each other. My father would not go to the market on Saturday when there were many more vendors and a much bigger selection. This frigid morning there were few shoppers, and those hardy souls that were there were making their purchases and leaving quickly. Most of the vendors were blowing on their hands, stamping their feet, and some had small fires burning in little grates.

As we walked down the aisles, he had one hand on my arm, his other hand on the guide stick. I described the wares that I saw—big oranges with their pungent smell, several varieties of apples, round leafy heads of iceberg lettuce. We approached tables that were laden with potatoes and onions. The Gray family, whom we knew from Joseph Avenue, took up a number of tables with their merchandise. My father asked Seymour Gray the price of a 50-pound bag of potatoes. He still believed in buying in large quantities, just as he had when he was in business.

"Potatoes are four dollars for fifty pounds." Seymour answered,

My father shook his head firmly and told Seymour, "It's too high."

"For you Sam, I'll make it three-fifty," answered Seymour. My father agreed to this adjustment. Hoisting the bag on his burly shoulder, Seymour carried the bag to our car. During this transaction I noticed that my hands were becoming numb, but we were not done with our buying expedition.

As we proceeded down an aisle I continued describing to my father the fruits and vegetables that were displayed. We stopped at a table stacked with citrus fruits. I handed my father one of the grapefruits so he could feel it and weigh it in his hands.

"This is a good size. Get a dozen," he requested.

I did as he asked, but I complained that my hands were turning to ice.

"You Americans, a liddle cold bodders you. Here, take my gloves." Feeling guilty I took his gloves and put them on over mine. First I checked his hands and found they were surprisingly warm. I felt less guilty as I pulled his gloves on.

Some of the vendors, themselves unable to keep warm and worried about their produce, were packing up. My father, however, wanted to check out the apples and celery. We hurried to an apple vendor while I noticed that now I was losing all sensation in my feet.

"There's hardly anyone left here, "I complained to my father in an injured tone of voice "Let's go home."

He insisted on buying apples and then grudgingly accompanied me to the car without the celery he wanted. I turned the car heater on full blast as we drove from the arctic air of the public market to Harriet's house. I unloaded the car first and then led my father into the house. He was looking forward to trying one of the apples and was pleased with the negotiated price of the potatoes. My hands and feet, though still tingling, were beginning to thaw.

After a quiet lunch we spent some time working on Braille. Neither one of us was ever to be very proficient, but for a time he tried to learn how to read the raised dots. His hands were still calloused and rough, but perhaps even more daunting was the fact that the English alphabet was not his native alphabet. He was willing to give it a try, so we struggled on.

I left him at the usual time, but made a brief detour to the supermarket where I could shop in warmth and comfort. It felt so good not to be freezing.

As I turned into the checkout I bumped into an acquaintance who stopped and looked at me with disapproval stamped all over her face. "Ruth, I saw you this morning with your father at the public market."

"Oh, did you? We were so busy shopping I didn't see you."

She smiled thinly and with reproach in her voice she asked gently, "Don't you think, Ruth, it was too cold to drag your father to the public market on a day like today?"

For a brief moment I didn't know what to say. Then I put a smile on my face and replied, "Oh, was it? Neither of us seemed to notice."

CHAPTER THIRTY

Work and Death

When he had his vision, my father's work had given him a sense of purpose and had provided a structure to his days. Now he turned again to his classes, listened to his talking books, went to prayer service twice a day, and talked to friends and relatives on the phone. He still hoped to find a job. I had started a part-time position in a library and had enrolled in a course with the intent of obtaining a master's degree in library science. We spent less time together. He was alone more, but he still retained his high spirits.

If you were to ask him how he felt, he would invariably reply "Tip top," and then he might ask, "I'm looking for a job. Do you know anyone who is looking for a good worker like me?"

The months rolled by, and soon another year had gone by, and then another, and another, and another. It was with great interest that my father listened one evening as Harriet read to him from the newsletter of the Association for the Blind. "Part-time cashier needed for the cafeteria at the Association." Harriet encouraged him to apply for the job. He did, and he got it. Thus, my father began his second career at the age of 78. More than fifty years earlier he had opened his own store on Joseph Avenue. He taught us to use the cash register and told us to "treat the customer right." Now he was delighted to be back behind a cash register dealing with customers again. He had no problem getting to work because I was able to drop him off on my way to school 20, where I had obtained a temporary position as school librarian for the academic year. A volunteer took him home.

My father's work as a cashier in the cafeteria involved adding—in his head, of course—the total of selections that the customer had recited to him. He would ring it up and give change if necessary. He sat with his arm partially covering the open cash register drawer so no one could reach into the till. He was able to identify coins by feel, but he had to ask what denomination of paper money was given to him. He then loudly repeated what the customer said so that those nearby could hear it, and he waved the money in the air at the same time. He thought by doing so, he would forestall anyone intentionally telling him he was getting a ten-dollar bill when it was really a five.

The Association for the Blind carried out a variety of training programs and served as a senior-citizen nutrition center. It also provided a sheltered workshop. A number of companies contracted out production work that could be completed by hiring those clients at the Association who were able and willing to work. Housed in a large, converted factory on Clinton Avenue, it contained several floors on which were teaching centers, kitchen facilities, a cafeteria, and the sheltered workshop. All those who used the facilities, or who worked there were required to find their own way from place to place without assistance. It was not meant for those who were unable to move about independently or who were unable to tend to their own needs. Everyone who worked there or came to the programs could buy food in the cafeteria.

My father talked to the customers as he worked. Some of the patrons were partially sighted; many had multiple handicaps. My father would try to entice them into trying things on the menu.

"Come on around, people," he would urge. "Come on around. I'm waiting for you. We've got the best coffee in town—fifteen cents a cup. Try the doughnuts. They are delicious. I can eat six at a time. We've got good cereal. Come on, people. We've got the goods; you've got the money. Try a fresh apple; an apple a day keeps the doctor away. Come on, people. Have your money ready. Come on around. I love you, people."

I asked the cafeteria supervisor what he thought about my father's ongoing monologue.

"It's great. Sam's talking is completely spontaneous and natural. His voice serves as a guide for the blind customers. It helps them find the cafeteria line more easily. His recital of various foods reminds them of the choices available. It's reassuring to our clientele to hear him," he replied.

My father handled over 300 transactions a day, and dealt with the blind and deaf, mentally retarded, old and young, and those with diverse disabilities. The assistant training supervisor, Sandy, said, "When Sam isn't talking, he is often humming to himself, and the other patrons soon find themselves humming the same tune."

I noticed when I was there, that often there was a consistent drone of humming all around me. She also remarked that the cash register had never added up as well at the end of the day as it did during my father's tenure.

Being back in the world of work brought my father untold satisfaction. He loved getting up each day and dressing for work. He enjoyed being with crowds of people. We all seemed to have come to terms, more or less, with life as it was. There were hard places to go through, difficulties and tensions to surmount, but we worked our way through it all. We seemed to have made an uneasy truce with fate.

That truce was shattered when my younger sister, Esther, died suddenly following a severe asthma attack in the early hours of a Sunday in October, 1978. Dan and I had just spent the previous evening at a dinner party at her house. We had left her and Jerry about midnight. There had been no indication that anything was seriously wrong, although I noticed that she was wheezing as she often did. When Jerry called us at six in the morning, to say Esther had just died, a numbness came over me—no crying or screaming—only a big emptiness.

My one clear thought was to comfort my father. Quickly, I dressed and drove to Harriet's house. When I entered, I thought I heard my father talking to someone. I found him standing alone in the middle of the living room, asking loudly of some Unseen Presence, "Why not me? I'm old and blind. Why her and not me?" I looked at him crying out from his world of darkness, and I thought to myself that this tragedy would crush his spirit; it would destroy him.

I was wrong, of course.

He sat silent and unshaven as throngs of friends and relatives came to offer their condolences during the week of Shiva (Jewish period of formal mourning). Through my own pain-glazed eyes I watched as he tried to pull himself together. He began answering the visitors' words of comfort. Each day during the week of Shiva he struggled to straighten his shoulders that were bowed with the heaviness of his grief. I listened as he tried to control the tremor in his voice. Paul, Esther's son was nineteen. Maureen was 23 and going through a divorce. Baby Kate, her daughter, was one year old. Maureen often sat on the floor next to my father, leaning against his leg. He would put his hand on her head, or pat her gently on the shoulder.

On the very last day of the week of Shiva, he and I were sitting on our low, hard chairs. There was a break in the stream of visitors who had been coming to pay condolence calls. I began to think and remember. I remembered Esther as a tiny baby, even then trying to breathe and play at the same time. One night, when she suffered an unusually severe attack, my mother summoned the doctor. He put Esther on our kitchen table so he could watch her because our bedroom was too dark and crowded. He sat next to her for hours, listening to her labored breathing. She suddenly stopped breathing. He quickly picked her up, and breathed into her mouth until somehow she began to breathe again.

There was so little to be done for asthma sufferers in those days. The one remedy that seemed to help Esther a little was inhaling the smoke from a green powder called Asthmador. To use it I needed the metal top of a coffee can. I poured a little bit of the green powder onto the coffee can top and lit a match to it. The powder would ignite and send up a heavy smoke whose scent would alleviate the wheezing after an hour or two.

I was about ten or eleven when Esther would come to me in the middle of the night instead of to my mother.

"I need the smoke," she would say breathlessly, I would quickly arise and go to her room, light a match to the powder, and we would settle down to wait for the smoke to fill the room. She would be sitting because it was too hard to breathe lying down. We would not talk together too much in the murk and haze because she needed all her energy to breathe. After an hour or two her breathing would be easier.

One winter day she had an asthma attack as we walked home from Number Nine School together. Although she was small and slight at six, she was too big for me to carry. I held her hand and covered her face with her scarf to protect her from the cold air. I wanted to get home in a hurry, but I knew we had to walk slowly. We stopped every few minutes so she could rest. I kept saying, "Only a little bit more," I kept saying. "We're getting there. It's not much further." When we finally got home, I delivered Esther to my mother and then burst into tears.

Nothing could keep Esther down for long. In school she was popular. Even in grammar school she had a circle of good friends who were always ready to go to movies, play Monopoly, roller skate, and have whatever fun they could devise. When she got to high school we called her "the party girl" because she was always ready to go when good times beckoned, even if it meant not doing her homework. Boys flocked to her, and I, four years older, was jealous. She was a great mimic and could reduce us to uncontrollable laughter with her imitations of people we knew. Her asthma attacks never abated, yet she refused to slow down or pay attention to them.

Of the four of us sisters, she and I argued the most. As teenagers we borrowed each other's clothes, and invariably, an argument would ensue. "You must have got a spot on my blouse," I yelled at her.

"It was there when I put it on," she yelled back.

"I am never going to let you borrow anything of mine ever again," I proclaimed and then flounced out of the room. For at least two days we would not borrow from each other. One of us would soon ask for a coveted sweater that the other had, and the cycle would begin again. During final exam week in her senior year of high school she confessed that she might not pass American History. The night before the exam she said, "I won't pass."

"You have to pass," I admonished, already practicing my later role as teacher. "You won't graduate if you don't pass." All night long I drilled her on the points I considered most important, making up mnemonic devices to promote accuracy.

"Give me three causes of the Civil War," I asked.

"SUE. Slavery, union—preservation of, economics."

"Very good, but you'll have to elaborate as much as possible. You're good at saying a little bit with a lot of words." I continued the pseudo quiz. "Name at least four pieces of New Deal legislation."

"FANS. Food, Drug, and Cosmetic Act, Agricultural Adjustment Act, National Labor Relations Act, Social Security Act."

"That's terrific. Just remember what they were for, too." Only when we both could not concentrate from exhaustion did we stop.

After her exam the next day she returned home from school, wearily shaking her head. "I don't know if I made it." A few days later she got the results. "I made it," she exulted.

"We both did," I felt compelled to remind her.

I thought of her on her wedding day, which took place two months after my own wedding. I bought a wedding dress that she and I both liked because we knew she would be wearing it only weeks after I wore it. I remembered her wheeling her children in their strollers. How my children loved to stay at her house when Dan and I would steal away for a weekend once in a while. She became a local celebrity because of her acting in various theater groups. We went to all the plays just to see her perform. On stage she could be funny or sad, serious or irreverent, but she always gave a stellar performance. I thought of all the Friday night dinners we had shared, the uproarious laughter that followed stories of her escapades, the times we had argued and then made up.

Sitting with my father in that still room on our last day of mourning, I was suddenly overcome by a sense of loss so sharp and overwhelming that I began to weep again. I tried to stifle my sobs so my father would not hear me, but he could tell I was crying.

"It's no use to cry too much," he said in a quiet voice. "You can't think of what was. We can't change it. We have to look ahead and do the best we can, and you have to be an example to your children of how to act."

I looked at his ravaged face and, I said to myself, *He is telling me the secret of how he has survived.*

Slowly we regrouped, retrenched, and sought to live a new kind of life, a life without Esther's sparkle. Those of us who knew my father knew what a struggle it was for him. Once again a light had gone out of his life forever.

CHAPTER THIRTY-ONE

Hawaii

All of us struggled to recover from the shock of Esther's death in our own way. It was a slow process, and by 1980, two years after Esther's death, our family had seen a number of changes. My father, now 80, had been working for two years as a cashier at the Association for the Blind. He relished being back in the world of work. Jerry was trying hard to put his life together. Their daughter, Maureen, was now a single mother after her divorce. We all doted on Maureen's little girl, Kate. Esther's son, Paul, a teenager when Esther died, sought comfort from his grandfather. My father was our example. Marcia, Harriet, and I made sure that Jerry, Paul, and Maureen knew that they could count on us. I babysat for little Kate as often as I could. Our Friday night dinners and Saturday lunches kept us closely in touch with each other. We kept our dinners traditional yet informal.

My father marshaled all his strength to reassemble the pieces of his life. While work was important to him, it was religion, so central a part of his life that helped him survive. Religious practice provided a framework for life to continue in its appointed pattern. The very first Friday after the week of formal mourning was finished, my sisters and I began preparations for our usual Friday night Sabbath meal.

"You're not going to have a big family dinner on Friday, are you?" a friend said to me. "You can't all be up to it with your sister dead only a week. Why don't you skip it this week?"

I was startled by her question. It had never occurred to me to skip our Sabbath meal. How could you skip the Sabbath? It was like saying "Let's skip the sunrise today; I don't feel like getting up." The Sabbath was there. It was immutable. My father would only feel worse if we did not prepare our Friday night dinner and midday meal on Saturday. We had been preparing our Sabbath meals together since my mother's death almost twenty years earlier. The first Friday after the formal week of mourning for Esther, we had our Sabbath dinner together, my sisters, our spouses, our children and the little great-grandchild.

We picked up our activities and routines, carefully choosing our individual routes to manage the new landscape of our lives. For my father it was a wrenching effort. He wept tearlessly every Friday before he recited the prayer over the wine. His voice broke, and he stopped until he could go on. We all stood silently around the table, waiting for him to regain control. I knew he never expected to outlive any of his children. I knew he missed Esther, her presence, her laughter, her jokes, her stories about the world of the theater. She had regaled us with countless anecdotes, some hilarious, some bizarre, told only as she could. We missed her. I felt the loss with a physical pain like a gnawing inside my chest. It was a hard time in every way for all of us.

We had not been on a family trip for seven years. Our first one in 1972 had included the most family members—eighteen of us. We were then our own tour group. On our next one in 1973 twelve of us had enjoyed the Jewish Highlights of Europe trip.

"I think it's time for another trip," my father suddenly said to me. "Find out where everyone wants to go." I perked up. My trip-planning skills were rusty from disuse after seven years, but it wouldn't take long to polish them up.

We knew it would be a difficult trip, our first without Esther, and the most diverse in age. My father was now eighty, and Kate almost three.

"Where does everyone want to go?" he asked me. I took a poll of all the family members to determine a place they'd always wanted to see. It surprised me that one place always came up—Hawaii. Could we manage it? We consulted our travel agent, and confirmed that we could manage a ten-day trip that covered three islands. Once more all the details about vacation times, work schedules, and school time for each one had to be checked. Fifteen of us left Rochester August 11, 1980, for what turned out to be a remarkably beautiful trip.

As we stepped off the plane on our first stop, Honolulu, a beautiful girl in a grass skirt greeted us warmly and put a lei around each of our necks as she planted kisses on our cheeks.

"They're glad to see us," my father said. "They like Americans."

"Father, they are Americans. We're all Americans."

The structure of our trips had become much looser. All the children, now young adults, spent more time on their own and at the beach. Each of us had time to explore what seemed most interesting or exciting. The museum lovers, the shoppers, the beachcombers, the sightseers, all grouped anew each day to enjoy various activities. We met almost every evening for dinner and exchanged stories of our day's adventures. There was always someone ready to watch the baby, have lunch with Grandfather, or walk along the beach at sunrise with a sleepless family member. We still changed rooms so my father could have the "best room." We still had our orientation sessions with my father when we first arrived at a hotel. The grandsons, and now Jerry, who was alone, took turns sharing a room with my father.

Everything about Hawaii was different, and all of us tried to convey to my father what we saw and felt. The weather was decidedly different. What a joy it was to wake up to blue skies, sunshine and warmth—how nice to escape the damp gray days of Rochester. We noticed, too, that the pace of life was slower. My father could tell how patient the sales people, the clerks, the hotel staff, the waiters and waitresses all were. There was none of the rushing about that we were used to.

I did not relinquish my role as entertainment chairperson easily. I kept trying to round everyone up for shows and sightseeing. "Hey, everybody, how about going to a pineapple plantation this afternoon?" I asked.

Some preferred to go to the beach. The shoppers hoped to find authentic Hawaiian shirts and other locally made items. in the boutiques and shops. I gave up on the plantation idea. One morning we went to the beach with Katie and played in the white sand. The next day I suggested we all go to the Kodak Hula Show. "It's free," I told everyone. "We'll see native dances and hear songs of the islands. Besides, Kodak's headquarters is in our hometown. Don't you think we should show our support?" A large group of us decided to go, and took a bus directly to the site which was a large field surrounded by bleachers.

Before finding seats Dan took pictures of the people wearing native dress. A woman dressed in a grass skirt, brightly flowered top, with a lei around her neck, came up to Dan and me and declared, "You are our winners for today. You are the lucky ones." We looked at her in bewilderment. We didn't know there was a competition going on. Where was the contest? How is it we won? What did we win?

The woman explained that for each show she and her staff look for a spectator who is using a Kodak camera. She was particularly pleased to choose Dan because he was bald. Part of the prize was a kiss on the top of the head. She preferred to kiss bald men because she didn't like to wind up with hair in her mouth. She placed a lei around Dan's neck and mine. Then she put a wreath of flowers on Dan's smooth shiny head. He reminded me of a Roman Emperor, or was it Bacchus? The other part of our prize was special seats for the show. Not for us, the bleachers. We had two seats right on the field close to the performers. Sitting in such seats we could view the show's exciting dances and music with special appreciation. I hoped the rest of the family were impressed with our short-lived fame.

With my father's encouragement our sightseeing in Honolulu included as much as we could comfortably do. The shoppers in the group had a splendid time going to one of the largest shopping malls in all of the United States. When we toured the Iolani Palace I said, "Father, this is the only palace on American soil." One night we went to a South Sea Spectacular, a dazzling show in the Bora Bora Room. My father enjoyed everything we did, listening as we described the shows we saw together, imagining the flowers and palm trees that lined the streets, the architecture, and the historic landmarks we toured. Our days were busy, but not hectic. We all took great pleasure walking along the beach, swimming, and listening to the waves. Always my father delighted in sharing it all with each of us.

From Honolulu we took a plane to the garden island of Kauai, a lush, tropical paradise, and the setting for the TV series, Fantasy Island. A picture of Ricardo Montalban was displayed in the lobby of our hotel. We were dazzled by the Coco Palms Resort Hotel, our home for three gorgeous days. I described to my father the opulence of the hotel and the luxury of our rooms. I was taken aback by the bathroom, particularly the sink, and I warned my father. "The bathroom sink is a big conch shell. It has jagged points all around. If you bend over the sink, one of those jagged edges could stab you in the throat. So don't bend over the sink to wash up by yourself." I couldn't help worrying that the sink might injure one of us. Each time I brushed my teeth or washed my face I measured carefully where I placed my face or hands.

We spent much of our time walking on the magnificent grounds, or along the beach. The waves were very powerful here, and we were mesmerized by the sight and sound of the pounding surf.

All of us enjoyed the food—succulent fruit, pineapple such as we had never had, fish that even my father, the expert, declared was unsurpassed for its taste, and always our meals were accompanied by careful attentive service. We passed up the luau (a pig roast—there was no such thing as a kosher pig), but each meal we had was a culinary delight. I dared to try a poi cocktail and loved it.

I took hula lessons and felt I was becoming most accomplished. No one else wanted to join me in this endeavor, but my father cheered me on. Every evening when shadows fell, torches were lit and the flames rose along the Coco Palms Tropical Lagoon following the Nightly Ceremony. Could our next island compare to this place?

It could and, in my eyes, it did. Once again we were overwhelmed by the natural beauty of our setting. Maui was a fitting end to our trip. The Royal Lahaina Hotel was perhaps even more luxurious. I was particularly glad we had ordinary sinks, and not those difficult and dangerous sea shells. My father enjoyed the beach, the walks among the trees and flowers. One day we took a trip in a glass-bottomed boat. Sometimes we took the hotel shuttle to a village that the shoppers found irresistible. One time some of us took my father to an ice cream parlor, the Royal Scoop, where my father could indulge in his favorite treat, a vanilla ice cream cone. On our last afternoon Dan and I saw a beautiful rainbow arching across the sky. My father was with us, and I described the colors to him and asked, "Do you think it means anything? Do you think it means good luck?"

He answered, "No question. It means we're all gonna have mazel." My father was pleased with the trip. He had swum in the Pacific surf, heard the music and the songs of the islands, smelled the tropical flowers, and listened to our descriptions of all we had seen and done. None of us was ready to leave when departure day arrived, but this time all of us, including my father, had a job to return to.

CHAPTER THIRTY-TWO

Nate

"I was so busy today, you can't imagine. We had a few specials, and everybody was buying. The boss told me I'm doing good."

My father's voice was full of pleasure as he described his workday to all of us. He went every day with great zest. I found myself hoping he would work at this job until the day he died—he loved it. Even after a day's work he still possessed the energy to pursue his other interests. Worship services were a top priority. Visiting friends and relatives was a favorite pastime. He chaffed at the need to depend on others for transportation, he who had always been the one to give a ride to others when needed.

He decided that he wanted to visit his old friend, Nate, who lived on the other side of town. My father felt confident that he could find his way to Nate's place using public transportation. Harriet pointed out that he would need to transfer to another bus downtown and locate the second bus stop. Then he would have to get off at his destination unaided. Everyone in the family vetoed the idea, foreseeing all kinds of possible problems. My father had at least three offers of a ride to visit Nate.

"Why can't your friend visit you?" I asked. "It would be much easier for him. He can see what he is doing."

My father answered, "My friend is afraid to take such a long bus ride."

Nothing further was said. A week later on a Sunday, Harriet came home to an empty house. Our father was nowhere to be seen. She called each of us, her voice shaking with anxiety, asking if we had seen Father. No one had any knowledge of his whereabouts.

"You don't suppose he took off to see his friend, do you?" I asked Harriet.

"He knew we would all try to stop him," she answered grimly "The Sunday bus schedule is so erratic—suppose someone tries to rob him or suppose he gets lost? How could he do this to us?"

We envisioned an accident or someone taking advantage of him. I wondered if she would soon get a call from the police reporting that my father had been found lost and wandering, or from a hospital telling her that he had been found hurt and bleeding.

In a short while my father called Harriet to announce that he was with his friend, Nate, and would someone come to pick him up and take him home. His voice was exuberant and happy.

Dan and I drove across town to pick up my father. We applauded his achievement, but explained that none of us wanted to ever again experience the worry and concern we had felt at his disappearance.

"You would stop me if I told you," My father replied. "I couldn't write a note so I thought, I'll just go."

He had found his way to the bus going downtown because we had taken walks that way a number of times. He got a bus transfer and was let off at Main and Clinton. A kindly stranger apparently took him to the second bus, which he boarded. He told the bus driver where he wanted to get off, and the driver called out his stop. When the bus arrived Nate was there to meet him.

They had a very fine visit. If my father thought that Nate would be inspired to take a bus trip to see him, he was mistaken. Nate remained too timid to take the trip. My father said with a note of superiority in his voice, "If I can do it, he can do it."

"Everybody's different," I said in defense of Nate. "He can't help it if he's afraid." I felt sorry for Nate, who had been a good friend when my father could see. A number of times he had gone with my father on shopping expeditions to the supermarket to help my father carry cartons of supermarket specials back to our store. My father and Nate continued their friendship by phone because my father didn't try to visit him again, and of course, Nate wouldn't dream of attempting such a long bus ride.

Although we had been shaken by my father's disappearance, we were proud and pleased for him. He refused to let our fears stop him from rising to the challenges he set for himself.

CHAPTER THIRTY-THREE

Roommates

"I didn't want a roommate," Randy, my nephew, was talking to me. "I wasn't ready for one. After all, I was only seven years old, and Grandpa was 72." I had asked him to have lunch with me, and we were reminiscing. He was now a young man in his twenties, and I had never asked him how he felt when my father went to live with his family and had moved into his room. I was surprised at myself for not talking to him long before.

"Didn't you ever resent his being there?" I asked.

"I knew something terrible had happened. My mother told me how Grandpa had been attacked in his grocery store and blinded, that all of you didn't think he should live alone anymore. We thought he would be with us for a little while, but he was my roommate for the first seven years that he lived with us."

Randy's words brought back those days of grief and shock. My father, at that time, a widower for over ten years, had never planned to live with any of his four daughters. He enjoyed taking care of his half of the two-family home he owned on Harvard Street. Mary came once a week to clean the house. He was strong and completely independent. All that changed when he was so brutally attacked.

"I knew we all had to pitch in and help," Randy continued. "My mother explained that we were the logical ones for him to live with first, because she was a nurse and knew how to help him. Besides, my room was big; I had an extra bed in my room, and it was better for him to have a boy for a roommate than a girl, like my sister."

"How did it work out?" I asked.

"Sometimes he would have nightmares at night and start screaming. He was reliving the whole attack. I'd wake up scared, but my mother would come running in to comfort him, and then she'd come to me. When I was a little older, I learned to calm him, and she didn't need to run in so much." It had never occurred to me before that Randy had had to wait to be comforted while Harriet first calmed my father before she turned her attention to her frightened son.

"You must have done a good job of helping him feel safe, because he was always in great spirits during the day," I said.

"At first it was hard for me to remember to put all my toys away so Grandpa wouldn't trip over them," Randy said. "I learned not to move anything in the room because he could get confused or lost if I did." I could picture seven-year-old Randy looking around his room to make sure everything was in the right place and that nothing was out of order.

He paused, his face thoughtful. "I saw how you and my aunts and uncles and cousins were all helping us, taking Grandpa out, going places with him, taking care of his affairs for him. I found out about family support then. I wanted to be part of our family effort to make life fun again, even if it meant we couldn't always do what we wanted to do."

He smiled when he said, "Sometimes I wouldn't get much sleep. He'd get up in the middle of the night to go to the bathroom. The banging and clacking of the guide stick against the furniture as he found his way would wake me up. Night and day were all the same to him. He had a talking clock, and many times he liked to check the time to see if he should get up. I'd hear a clipped voice announce, 'The time is three A.M.' Other times I'd hear a crinkling sound in the night. I would be in a deep sleep, and as I was waking up, I tried to figure out what was crinkling. When I got my eyes open and looked around I'd see Grandpa, lying in bed, unwrapping a piece of hard candy. He loved sour balls and took a bag to bed with him pretty often. Each piece was individually wrapped." Randy laughed. "I didn't get upset about it. He wanted his candy. Besides," he paused and said softly, "I loved him."

As we left the restaurant I put my hand on my nephew's shoulder. "You know what, Randy? I'll bet you can sleep through almost anything now."

They were roommates for almost eight years. When Randy was about 14 years old he wanted a room of his own. He asked Harriet and Bob, who agreed that Randy was ready for his own space. They suggested to my father that he might like a different room to sleep in. Their house had a small sun porch downstairs. They thought the room could be converted into a bedroom and a powder room. Harriet asked my father if he would split the cost of the remodeling with them.

"Why do we need to do this?" My father asked after thinking about it. "Randy never bothers me."

Bob said diplomatically, "Randy likes to play music in his room. Sometimes he asks a friend over so they can listen together. He doesn't like to disturb you."

My father laughed. "Don't worry about me. I don't see him. My ears are not so good anymore, so I don't hear him. He can do whatever he wants. It won't bother me." Harriet explained again that Randy needed his room back, and the downstairs location was better for my father. He would have his own room and bathroom and no longer need to go up and down the stairs so much. He kept saying the present arrangement was fine.

After several months, Harriet asked me if I could talk to my father. "Maybe you can persuade him that it's a good idea."

I took my father aside. "Father, when you were growing up, the nine people in your family slept in two rooms. Even when I was growing up, I shared not only a room, but a bed with Marcia, and for a while Harriet in her crib, was in the room with us, even though she was eight years old. Luckily she wasn't a great big girl, but that crib was pretty tight for her. Nowadays nobody does that unless they absolutely have to. As long as you can afford to have a downstairs room to yourself I think it would make your life easier and make Randy happy." He finally agreed, although he probably thought it a big indulgence at first.

He grew to enjoy his own room with its adjacent bathroom. "Why don't you put in a bathroom downstairs in your house?" he asked me. "I'll help you."

"Thank you, Father, but we already have one." My father was pleased.

CHAPTER THIRTY-FOUR

Benelux

The pattern of my father's days was satisfying—work, prayer services, visits to friends, Friday night dinners, and always time with all the family. Busy as he was with his work and activities, he still thought about taking trips. It was now 1983, three years since our last family trip, and my father suggested that I look into another one

Twelve of the family were able to go. Katie, Maureen's daughter, was now six, and my father was eighty-three. My father urged me to find a tour that would cover several countries

"Let's see a lot of countries. Let's get our money's wurt," he said. We decided on a trip called the Benelux tour, that included Belgium, the Netherlands, Liechtenstein and Luxembourg, as well as stops in France, Germany and England. Seven countries in eight days. Weren't we sure to get our money's worth? I felt compelled to follow my father's wishes, but I had qualms about the trip. Little did we know what such a pace entailed. It was a trip of mishaps and mistakes from the beginning. Harriet and Bob admitted that they didn't really recover for weeks.

I was tired before the trip began. We had to be at the airport by six-fifteen in the morning so we could depart for New York City by seven-ten. Harriet, our nurse, and Bob, our pharmacist, always had a large first aid kit with them on every trip. I felt safe traveling with them.

Harriet was dabbing Katie's ears with an alcohol-soaked cotton ball. Kate had had her ears pierced recently. "Your ears will feel much better very soon," she said soothingly. The rest of us were milling about. I tried to comfort Katie and to prod the sleepiest-looking members of the group into a more alert frame of mind now that I was wide awake.

My father was impatient as ever. "When are we leaving?" he kept asking whoever was nearby. He would say, "Let's keep moving. Why are we standing still?"

"There's no place to go, Father. We have to wait for the plane," Marcia answered. Our flight to New York landed just in time for us to make our connection. We raced through La Guardia, my father leading the pack and boarding first, with Harriet at his side. The flight to London was punctuated by our walks up and down the aisle, all of us checking on Katie and my father. In London we were met by our guide, who took us to our hotel by bus.

As soon as we each had our room assignments we were, as usual, running in and out of each other's rooms trying to figure out which should be my father's room. We were also sorting our luggage, which the bus driver had brought in and dumped in the lobby.

Harriet, looking distracted, asked, "Has anyone seen Bob's and my suitcase?" We discovered that their luggage was nowhere to be found. They wore the same clothes on the whole trip. Of course they spent more time than anyone else washing out their clothes. They spent valuable time going to the airline office to for fill out reports for their luggage. They also needed time to buy some underwear in Amsterdam. At one point their luggage did arrive in Brussels before we did, but an indifferent hotel clerk sent it back to Amsterdam, never bothering to verify that we would arrive shortly after their luggage left. Not until the second-to-last day of the trip did their suitcase catch up with them. We were never in one place long enough.

We had to be up very early every morning. Because of our pace, much of what we did was a blur. Holland enchanted us with its windmills, canals, magnificent flower auction and the Rijksmuseum. We were charmed by the story-book countryside of Germany. One of our more peaceful moments came when we glided down the Rhine

River on a ferry boat. Gazing at the countryside as we floated past, we saw castles, houses with beautifully tended flower boxes at the windows, and trains winding through the mountainside in the distance. All this we described to my father, trying to capture for him our appreciation of the unfolding landscape.

"It looks like a picture postcard," I told him.

"I think I saw scenes like this in a book I had," Maureen added.

For much of the time, however, we were on a bus. As our bus rolled along, I overheard Judy, my daughter, ask David, my son, "Where are we?"

David peered out the window at road signs in a foreign language he did not recognize, and finally gave her his best advice. "Figure out what day of the week this is, and then look on Mom's itinerary or ask the bus driver.

Some hours later the bus driver announced, "We are approaching Paris."

It had been ten years since we had been in Paris. Dan and I wanted to revisit the Louvre, see Montmartre for the first time and all of us hoped to walk everywhere and enjoy more of this city. On the metro the next day Bob lost his travelers checks to a pickpocket. He and Harriet spent even more precious time at the American Express Office making out additional reports.

Our pace did not slacken. "I'm tired," said Katie, and so were the rest of us.

Our father, for the first time, admitted that he needed more time to rest. Sometimes he preferred not to go with us.

"You go," he said. "I'm glad to lie down. I want you should all see everything and have a good time together." We followed his wishes, knowing he could find his way around his room while we were gone.

When we returned to London, the bus dropped us off at a seedy-looking hotel where we all disembarked only to find that no one was expecting us. It turned out to be the wrong hotel. After some phone calls another bus soon picked us up and took us to a grander hotel. In the lobby we rubbed elbows with Arabs in native dress, dark-eyed women with veils covering their faces, Africans in brightly colored garb, Asian families, and little children of every hue and description running about.

"Isn't this cosmopolitan and exciting?" we told each other. "Look at all the adorable children."

That evening I arranged for everyone to see *Singin' in the Rain* at the Palladium. We walked to the bus stop. While we waited Bob dropped his wallet. Before he could bend over to pick it up, an ill-clad man nearby rushed over, grabbed the wallet from the ground, and quickly dashed away. The performance of the musical was excellent, but a pall was cast over us as we thought of the stolen wallet.

During the night our much-needed sleep was disrupted several times by the harsh clanging of the fire alarm bell. It seemed that some of the adorable children we had seen running about the lobby when we arrived felt it would be fun to pull the fire alarm. The first time we all ran down to the lobby, frightened. We were widely dispersed through the twenty-three floors of the hotel; our request to be placed closer together, denied. When the fire alarm bell clanged us all awake in the middle of the night, Harriet ran up several flights to my father's room to make sure he and the boys were up and out. The second fire alarm found us less inclined to panic, and the third time a large number of hotel guests never even responded.

Since the next day was our last day, we all went in various directions. "Dan and I must go to the British Museum again," I said.

Harriet and Bob planned to go to the police station as early as possible to make out a report on the stolen wallet. "After the police station we're going to Fortnum and Mason's," said Harriet. "Marcia and Father are going with us."

Jerry, Maureen, Paul and Katie planned to go to the London Zoo. "Katie is going to love it," Maureen predicted. Before separating we set the time for our last dinner together. We knew we would, as usual, have to be up very early in the morning.

At dinner that night, everyone agreed the trip had been too hectic, almost frenetic, and had given us no time for rest or reflection. I missed what I called absorbing time, a space of time needed to get a feel of the locale. Especially with a group such as ours we needed more time than most to make plans for the day. We simply had needed more time. Maureen remarked that our trip had had some fine moments, but she added, "The pace was too fast for us. If we take another trip let's not try to cover so much ground in such a short time."

Katie said, "How about not doing more than five countries in a week next time?"

CHAPTER THIRTY-FIVE

Leaving Work

He was so happy to be going to work every day. The rhythm of his life suited him. He had worked from the time he was a child of ten. It had always been an essential part of him. Maybe now it served to make him feel more whole, less maimed.

He was ebullient when I took him home. He was absorbed and challenged by his work, and he thrived on it. He made less than minimum wage because his work was considered "sheltered employment." He joked about not making enough money to cover expenses, but the intrinsic value far outweighed any monetary consideration.

Every morning I picked my father up a little before seven-thirty. He had already been up since five o'clock, said his morning prayers, eaten his self-prepared breakfast, and dressed himself in the clothes that Harriet had set out the night before. He was usually at the door waiting for me. At the Association he handled the breakfast shift, the coffee break, and the lunch hour. After work I took him home. Sometimes he had a ceramics class in the afternoon or some other activity. He enjoyed being busy, but the highlight of his weekday was his work.

When my work changed, and I could no longer take him, the Lift Line took him to the Association and brought him home. When he came home after lunch he emptied his pockets of the plastic spoons and forks he had slipped into his pockets. He also took out the clean paper napkins and little packets of sugar.

"Father, why are you taking these things from the Association and bringing them home?"

"I'm entitled to eat lunch there, but I don't," he answered. "I figure I can take these things home instead. Maybe you can use them."

I noticed that he even took things from Harriet's supper table to put into his pockets. Sometimes he offered me an orange or apple that he had squirreled away. I tried to dissuade him, but he felt it was perfectly acceptable. It was amazing how many apples and oranges he was able to hide in his pockets. My sister, Harriet, at that time a nurse at Strong Memorial Hospital, recounted a story revealing how adept he had become at it.

"One time Father did not feel well at his ceramics class at the Art Gallery and fainted. The Gallery sent him to Strong by ambulance. I was alerted that my father was being brought into emergency, and I quickly arranged to meet him there. I didn't know if he had a serious problem. I was waiting for him when he was brought in on a stretcher. I could hear him saying that he was perfectly all right, that nothing was wrong with him, he could walk in, why was he wasting time lying on a stretcher? I went to him and assured him that it was best to check that there was no big problem. I told him a brief examination would not take too much of his time. As I helped him take off his shirt and jacket, apples and oranges fell to the floor and began rolling in all directions, along with little sealed packages of a dessert of some kind. I'm looking at everything rolling around the floor, and I don't know what to say. Maybe my colleagues think he doesn't get enough to eat at home.

"'I think he must be hungry,' I tell the doctor and other nurses.

"'Harriet, pick everything up. I don't want to lose anything,' he says to me.

"We can laugh now, but I was so embarrassed then," Harriet said. Neither Harriet nor I could change this habit. I thought of his years of want and deprivation. Did it make him feel secure to have something in his pockets to eat? I didn't argue with him. I didn't want anything to upset him, and I knew it would do no good. I was unbelievably happy for him, because although he was blind, every day he went off to do work that he enjoyed and was proud of.

His work was such a joy to him that I found myself hoping again that he could work until he died peacefully in his sleep. I felt guilty thinking about death, but now that I could see how much it meant to him to be back in the world of work I couldn't imagine how he could be without it.

For eight years he rarely missed a day except for family trips and religious holidays. At the age of 85 he was still eager to keep working. Because I was lulled into a sense of security about my father's work, I really thought it would go on for his lifetime. It was a shock when someone from the Association called to say that my father was slowing down in handling his customers. The cafeteria line was growing too long. It was backing up, and they needed it to move faster. They felt my father could not keep up the necessary pace. My sisters and I talked over what to do or say. How should we handle the situation? We arranged to meet with his supervisor.

The staff was kind. They listened to our concerns and understood.

"We can find something else for him to do, but he can't stay as cashier," the supervisor said.

Grateful that there was another spot for him, we accepted the offer for my father.

He was not aware of his diminishing pace or of our discussions with the staff. My sisters and I told him that the cafeteria job was needed for someone else and that he would henceforth be doing a different job— stripping film.

My father found stripping film much less enjoyable. He was not talking to people in his new job. He missed that interaction. The work itself was not too difficult for him. He had to meet certain targets which he came close to meeting, sometimes even exceeding them, but another problem soon became apparent. From the very beginning of his time at the Association we had known that workers needed to be able to move about independently. Now, my father could not find his way from his new work station to the bathroom or to the cafeteria for his break. The staff had worked with him, and he'd had the usual training, but he could not learn the route. I asked the supervisor if my sisters and I could work with him, taking extra time to teach him the route. The supervisor agreed, asking only that we teach him during slow hours when we would not be disrupting large numbers of people moving about. I was sure we could teach my father the new route. I had seen the route, and I knew it was not complicated.

I told my sisters, "All three of us are very good teachers, aren't we? Harriet teaches nurses how to be good nurses. Marcia and I are patient and clear when we talk to little kids. By the time we're done going over this with him, he'll be able to do this route better than anyone."

We had promised not to interfere with the busy time. Late in the afternoon when few people were there we each took turns on different days going back to the Association with him. I went over and over the route. The next day Harriet went over the route, and Marcia the following day. We took turns for several weeks. He could not learn the route. He kept getting lost. He could not find his way alone. He would have to give up working. How were we to tell him? What could we say that would not damage his self-esteem? He would no longer be able to get up each day, secure in the certainty that his work awaited him, that he was needed at his job, that the framework of his day involved productive, paying work.

Again Marcia, Harriet and I met with the supervisor and an assistant to discuss our dilemma—how do we handle this? The Association staff had been understanding in their effort to keep him working, and when that proved impossible, they resolved to make his departure as happy as they could. My sisters and I had a plan that we hoped would help lessen the pain of his last days of work. We explained to the staff that we had a trip coming up. That winter, at my father's urging, we had started to talk about a trip to Scandinavia. We had already finished our usual discussions and preliminary research concerning itineraries, prices, and schedules. By early spring we had chosen a tour, and August 10 was our departure date. A larger number of family members had decided to go, and I was happy so many of us would be together on another journey to see the world. My father was making suggestions about what to take, and was as excited as all of us about visiting

Denmark and Sweden. We felt it would be good for him to work until the trip. The supervisor said they would allow him to do that. After the trip the supervisor said that the Association staff would make a retirement party for him, and he would have that to look forward to. With their help we orchestrated my father's last days as a working man. Most importantly, my father had to be urged to retire. I broached the subject directly.

"Father," I told him several weeks before our trip, "I think you should retire."

"Why?"

"I think you've worked long enough. You're 85, and it's time to give someone else a turn."

All of us carried on this kind of conversation with him. He seemed to give it some thought—but not enough.

We continued our conversations. "You don't really need the extra money, Father. Some people need it more than you do. They need money for food and clothing. Some of these younger blind people don't have very much put away. Maybe they've been blind since birth."

That made him pause. I felt he was remembering his days of poverty.

I kept talking. " Listen to me, Father. The Association has to help the blind people get along on their own. They know you can manage without your salary. Maybe that's why they moved you around. Why not retire while you're ahead, before they tell you they need your job for someone else? You can be the one to let another person have an opportunity that could make a big difference."

"All right," he said. "I'll retire."

"Let's get busy and work on getting our trip in order. We'll be leaving soon," I reminded him.

We left on August 10, 1985, in the afternoon and landed in Copenhagen the next morning at eight.

CHAPTER THIRTY-SIX

Scandinavia

"Wonderful, wonderful Copenhagen, friendly old girl of the sea," I sang softly as we rode the bus to our hotel. Never had I thought I would see Denmark. When I was a child our family had done very little traveling. A motor trip to Utica, New York, to see cousins was a major journey and seemed to take days of preparation. I didn't think any of us could get tired of taking trips with my father. Each new city brought us anticipation and excitement. The days of cleaning fish seemed eons ago.

After our overnight flight we arrived at our hotel a little before nine in the morning. To my dismay, we were told that our rooms would not be available until 1:30 or 2:00 in the afternoon. Only one room was ready, and out of deference to my father's 85 years, we insisted he take it to get some rest. He invited us all into the room, and everyone found a spot to lie down or curl up. Several of the younger members lay on the floor, some draped themselves over a couple of stuffed chairs. Someone stretched out at the foot of my father's bed. We kept our voices low and did not disturb my father, who could sleep anywhere.

By mid-afternoon we had chosen the "right" room for my father, finished the orientation, and were set to go. In a group, we all headed for Tivoli Gardens. Across the street from the entrance Harriet spotted a restaurant. She said, "Let's eat before we go in. I'm starving. We haven't had much to eat all day."

It was a pleasant eating place we had chosen, and we all sat around some tables the waiter had helped us push together. Harriet read to my father the items on the menu that she thought he would relish. My father chose herring and thoroughly enjoyed it. Our dinner was all the more festive because David and Shelley were celebrating their first wedding anniversary. When we had finished our dinner and were all ready to enter the Tivoli Garden, Harriet and Bob returned to the hotel with my father. He was already too tired to do more. He needed to go to bed.

The rest of us continued into Tivoli Garden and were dazzled by the brilliantly colored lights. We hardly knew where to look first. There were all kinds of rides, restaurants, concerts, shows, shooting galleries, games of chance, and fireworks. As I walked through the park I wished my father had been with us. He would have enjoyed the excitement.

The next morning, all of us, including my father, were up early and ready for our three-hour sight-seeing bus tour of Copenhagen. The guide pointed out landmarks and told us historical anecdotes, but we added our own comments for my father's benefit. He always enjoyed hearing the descriptions of what we were seeing. When it was over we all had lunch together, and then the others dispersed to go shopping and sight seeing, while Dan and I returned to the hotel with my father, who wanted to lie down for a while.

When I stopped by his room a little later he asked, "Do you think we could go to a synagogue? I would like to go to services."

"I'll find out if there's a synagogue we can get to," I told him.

My queries in the lobby brought forth the necessary information and directions to the nearest synagogue. Paul, my nephew, and Kate, my six year old great-niece, were back from their shopping expedition and wanted to go with us. After a short cab ride we arrived at a beautiful, modern synagogue. We participated in the service, knowing that if we had been back in Rochester, we would have been reciting the same words in the prayer service. The members of the congregation were very security conscious because a bomb had exploded and damaged the synagogue a couple of weeks earlier.

People ushered us out of the building immediately after the service saying, "We still don't feel safe here."

It was close to dinner time, and a member of the congregation kindly offered to take us to a kosher restaurant in the Jewish Community Center. We squeezed ourselves into his tiny Volkswagen. Our thoughtful acquaintance dropped us off at the JCC and instructed us about the intricacies of finding the doorbell which was in a partially hidden spot. We followed his advice carefully. In answer to the ringing bell, the door slowly opened.

A young man looked all five of us over. He invited us into a simple, almost austere, dining room. "We are all still upset over the bomb, and we are being extra careful," our waiter told us, as he handed us the menu. "We worry that all places with Jewish connections might still be a target. That's why we're so nervous and edgy."

Looking over the menu I noticed several favorites—chicken fricassee, potato latkes, cholent, stuffed kishke. My father enjoyed his chicken soup and chicken, the first and only time he had meat on the trip. It was dark when we left. We took a cab back to our hotel, and as soon as I paid the cab driver I took my father to his room. He was too tired to do anything but go to bed. When he was comfortably settled, Dan and I joined the others in the lounge. It was here we all talked together, exchanged stories of our various adventures, and made some plans for the following days.

The next morning all of us took a boat ride in the harbor and looked at the little mermaid who sat near the shore. One evening all of us, including my father, went to a one-ring circus with amazing acrobats, trapeze artists, jugglers, and a bear riding a bicycle. I told him, "There's a beautiful lady swinging on the trapeze way up in the air holding on by her teeth—not her hands, Father—only her teeth."

He shook his head back and forth in wonderment. "Oombelievable," he said.

"Oh, Father, there's a great big brown bear riding a bicycle. The bear seems to be in a bad mood. It looks like he's not following instructions."

"How can you tell?" he asked.

"A small little lady, probably the trainer, is running next to him pointing at something, like she wants him to do a trick, but the bear keeps waving a paw at her as though he wants to push her hand away."

Her voice rising with excitement, Maureen added, "Now she's moved a little away from the bear, and she's not pointing at him anymore. Oh, oh, it looks like the bear act is over. A couple of people are walking off with him. I think he's not a happy bear tonight, and nobody wants to force him to do anything. If he really got upset he might try to attack somebody."

I saw him raking the air with his paw even as he walked off. My father shook his head knowingly, as though he were experienced in the ways of animals, and said, "A wild animal is always a wild animal."

Out came a group of lithe, good-looking performers. As we described the human pyramids, the handsprings and somersaults of the acrobats, my father asked, "Is everybody having a good time?"

"We're having a wonderful time. I don't think any of us has seen a circus like this."

The next day at Elsinore, my father walked slowly as we described where we were. We alternated keeping him company so that eventually everyone could explore everything. We each told my father about our impressions of the magnificent castle. He was very tired when we returned to our hotel and went to bed after a light meal that we brought to his room. That night we had to pack and be ready to leave early in the morning.

The next day, after breakfast, we boarded a train that rolled onto a ferry for the eight-hour trip to Stockholm. The guide that we expected to meet at the station didn't show up.

"Why isn't anyone here?" asked Maureen.

"Where do we go?" asked Paul. "And how do we get there?"

"Who made these arrangements? I think we should call our travel agent back in Rochester and complain," said someone else.

What had gone wrong? I thought we had taken care of every possible problem.

My father interrupted my thoughts, announcing, "I have to go to the men's room."

"Are there any men available to take Father to the bathroom?" asked Harriet, raising her voice above the general hum. "I don't think it's on this level. You might have to find the elevator or an escalator."

After I made several phone calls, a bus was sent to pick us up and take us to our hotel. By the time we had looked to see which room was best for my father and had done our orientation with him, it was dinner time. After a splendid meal, my father went to bed, but the rest of us went out to walk and breathe the air of Stockholm.

Our days were filled with the sights we chose to see and the activities each of us enjoyed—sometimes together, sometimes separately. My father either went with one of us or said he wanted to rest. We made sure that there was always someone to have lunch with him and take a little walk. All of us went to Skanson together and kept up a running commentary for him about this outdoor recreated village.

"Father," I told him, "We are in Europe's oldest outdoor museum. There are over 150 old houses and buildings from all over Sweden right here. We've got something like this at home, only its not so big or so old as this one." On another day all of us were awed by the Wasa Museum, the museum that displayed actual ships that had been brought up from the floor of the ocean.

"Listen everybody," I addressed the group, "Can you believe that this warship, the Wasa, sank after twenty minutes into its maiden voyage in 1628? Everybody on it died. There it lay for 333 years. Then it was finally raised. It's the best preserved ship of its kind." I finished reading from the tour book and closed it, satisfied that I had done my duty as tour guide.

We took a bus tour of Stockholm and were dropped off at Old Town—centuries old. The Palace contained an Armory in the basement, where Paul and I walked around looking at the weaponry of long ago.

On our last night we had dinner at the Grand Hotel, a beautiful hotel that lived up to its name. It was known for its Swedish smorgasbord. Actually none of us had the smorgasbord. As we talked and laughed that last night at the long table in the elegant dining room, I thought of my father's oft repeated words, "Travel is educational." We had, indeed, become acquainted with another culture—its people so blonde and tall, its seafaring history, the foods, but we had learned about ourselves as well. I had a powerful sense of family, of responsibility assumed and shared, a willingness to accommodate to the needs of the moment. We had not known, until this trip, how much my father's strength had diminished. He walked more slowly, tired so much more quickly, needed more help. Now, for the first time, we understood what the people at the Association had meant.

After dinner a few family members forbade anyone to leave our table. There was some whispering and discussion going on among the group. Maureen, apparently the spokesperson for everyone, stood up and announced, "Aunt Ruth, we have a gift for you. All of us want you to know we appreciate all you have done as our tour arranger. You have our gratitude, and here is our token of appreciation."

She handed me a package. I unwrapped the gift and found a handbag I had admired on a shopping expedition the day before—gray suede with a handle of gray leather. I was sitting next to my father. I put my hand on his, and I looked around me at the pleased faces of the people I loved. We were coming to the end of another trip. They were the ones who had made all the trips a success. Their flexibility, their ever present readiness to change their own plans for the good of the group had made it possible to travel everywhere together. In each trip some parts were funny, or poignant, or difficult, but we had found ways to work out the problems. Did they know the meaning of what we had all shared? At that moment, I had feelings I knew I could not express. Pressing my father's hand, I looked at everyone and said, "Thank you all very much for this gift. I loved being our tour organizer, and I'm ready to go again whenever you are."

CHAPTER THIRTY-SEVEN

First Cruise

"It's time to take another trip." Although my father was now eighty-six years old and not as sure about finding his way, he was still eager to "see" the world. The patriarch of our family, he had not lost his drive to keep us doing things together.

"Talk to the family. Find out where they want to go," he said to me, the self-proclaimed chief of family-trip planning. "And we don't want to go to the same places we were before," he added. I told him we could return to London or Paris or Madrid, because there was so much to do and see in those cities.

"No, let's go someplace new," he insisted. But our choices were not so wide as my father supposed. On our most recent trip to Scandinavia, we were all shocked at my father's diminished energy and his loss of stamina.

Harriet, warned, "We want a trip with a minimum of walking or sight seeing for him. You can all see how quickly he tires these days." She knew better than any of us what he could do, but I didn't want to know that he could no longer lead the pack with his loud voice booming, "C'mon everybody, let's keep moving." He had been tireless when we first began taking our trips together in 1972.

"Where haven't we been that would not be too expensive, that would not involve too much walking, and that would be exciting?" I asked.

Someone suggested a Caribbean cruise, and it seemed like a perfect solution. My father insisted we check with the rabbi to see if traveling on the ship on the Sabbath was acceptable by religious law.

The rabbi said, "If the ship is already in motion then it's all right to be on the cruise. You can't start or stop your trip on the Sabbath."

On a cloudless day in August, twelve of us stood on the deck of the *Song of America* and waved good-bye to strangers on the receding Florida shore. I gazed out at the sea and felt that I was taking part in a movie. I always did on our trips. Had I ever dreamed as I cleaned fish and picked scales out of my hair, that one day I would be cruising on a luxury liner? I remembered that years before, in our neighborhood movie theater, I had watched as Fred Astaire and Ginger Rogers danced on board just such a ship. Now I, too, was living the life of the rich and famous. When I shared my feelings of wonder and amazement with my father, he always agreed and said in his inimitable English, "It's oombelievable."

Within the hour of boarding the ship a loud voice over the ship's public address system informed us that a boat drill was to be held very soon. Harriet went to my father's stateroom and helped him into his life jacket. He made it to the deck with her assistance. There on deck we all had our picture taken by the ship's photographer. The ubiquitous photographers were busy taking pictures at every turn—when we boarded ship, ate dinner, or simply walked the deck. Years later I still feel the pleasure emanating from the pictures, pleasure at being together and embarking on an exciting trip.

That night at our family meeting, we decided that whenever we docked at a port, the sons-in-law or the grandsons, hardy and strong, would help my father off the ship. Some of us would then go off sightseeing, and some would stay with him.

The days were sunny and warm. My father loved the water, and the ship's pool was inviting. He had never learned to swim properly, but he found pleasure in doing swimming strokes and ducking under the water. Harriet usually took him to the pool, and often Randy, Gail, Maureen, and her husband, Bill, joined them to swim or splash in the cool water under a hot sun. Some of us chose to have lunch with him on specific days, others walked around the deck with him and often helped him at lunch, too. Paul and Randy took turns sharing a room with their grandfather. A night in Grandfather's room meant a night of very fitful sleep.

We all enjoyed the lavish breakfasts, delicious lunches, elegant dinners, and the dazzling midnight buffets. Often a few of us indulged in the afternoon snack as well. At dinner we all ate together, dressed in our best, and compared notes on our various activities. I took my father to breakfast one morning and was glad to see how much he relished the food.

"I like these buns. They are very good. Take one for me to eat later," he said.

"Father, I don't think the captain would like us to take food back. I don't see anybody doing that. Besides, there's twenty-four-hour room service. That means we can call up the kitchen from the cabin and order whatever we want anytime of day or night. The waiter brings it right away."

"We don't need to call anybody. Take a banana, too," he added. We paid plenty for it. Just put it in your pocket."

"I don't have a pocket, Father. Besides, there's icing on the bun. If I had a pocket it would get full of crumbs and icing." I paused and looked at his face. He was not pleased with my reluctance to help him.

" All right," I gave in. "I'll take a napkin and wrap it around the bun and the banana."

He took my arm as we rose from the table. As we walked to the door the head steward approached us and said gently to me, " Please don't take any food out of the dining room. It's not necessary. You can order anything you want from your cabin."

I could feel myself flush with embarrassment. "I'm sorry. We didn't know," I said.

My father and I left the dining room in silence. We had both tacitly decided a long time ago we would not waste time with recriminations. We took a stroll around the deck as I described the sea and the sky. I told him about some of the passengers I observed and the smartly dressed staff. He listened to the sounds of voices around him, felt the breeze, and smelled the sea air. Through all our eyes he saw what we saw.

On Friday night, we discovered that there were Sabbath services on board for those of the Jewish faith, lead by the emcee of the ship's nightly entertainment, which was usually a musical revue.

The service was far too short and abbreviated for my father. I thought it was a fine length. I never minded a short service. The emcee had a pleasant enough voice for singing songs like "You Made Me Love You," but it lacked something for chanting the prayers. It was nice meeting the others at the service, and I had a good time, but my father was disappointed.

"That's not a Shabbos service," he complained.

Most of the time, though, he was happy and enjoyed doing everything. When we arrived at Nassau, Dan and I and my father walked off the gangplank straight into the heart of the colorful city. We sat on a bench in the park, and I described the scene to my father—the ship close by in the water, the sun shining on the busy street, the park with its tropical trees and flowers. We told him about the policeman directing traffic, who wore a white helmet, a dark uniform with gold buttons and white gloves. He moved with grace and precision, almost like a ballet dancer, as he turned and motioned with his hands to the lines of traffic, indicating with a wave when to move.

San Juan posed problems for us. My father wanted to get off at this port of call, but it was far more difficult than we had anticipated. There was a rope ladder to descend and a long walk on the wharf, but even with Dan above him and Bob below, assisting him down the rope, my father almost fell. When he finally got down, he was breathing hard and beads of perspiration glistened on his upper lip and forehead. He was too tired to do anything but sit down on the nearest bench. On our return to the ship we spoke to the officers, and my father was allowed to board through an entrance not usually used for passengers. He was exhausted when we got back. With a little extra rest he perked up, but we knew he had made a tremendous effort for us.

Each night he told us he preferred to go to bed early, but urged everyone to see the evening's entertainment.

If I came to check on him in his cabin, he invariably asked, "Is everybody having a good time?"

"Everyone is having a wonderful time, Father. We love every minute. We'll all remember this forever." I knew I was telling him what he wanted to hear, but I also knew it was the truth.

At the midnight buffet, Ice sculptures in the shape of dolphins, mermaids, or fanciful fish adorned the tables. Magnificent desserts of every description, raw vegetables shaped into flowers—an endless variety of food enticed the most disciplined weight watcher. We always described the beauty of the spread tables as well as the abundance and the excellence of the food to my father the next day. I wondered if he thought of the times so long ago in Europe when he was always hungry, and when people would kill for food.

At dinner on our last night together we all toasted our first cruise together.

"We'll go again next year," he promised. He raised his glass of wine and said, "L'chaim" (to life).

CHAPTER THIRTY-EIGHT

Nursing Home Decision

It was very hard for me to see how much slower he walked. He paused after every four or five steps to catch his breath. Walking home from Sabbath services on Saturday was so difficult for him that he could hardly speak when he arrived at Harriet's house. (As an observant Jew he never drove on the Sabbath.) Harriet argued with him about not going to services on Saturday. It did not take much arguing, but he needed to feel he was doing her a favor by not going

"Father, you can hop a ride with me. I'll drive you over any Saturday you want to go," I said

He laughed at my audacity for suggesting such a thing. "I never did before," he answered, "and I'm not going to start now."

Soon he could no longer find his way around Harriet's house. For almost fifteen years he had walked from room to room with confidence and ease. Now Harriet found him exhausted from the effort of trying to locate his room. He would walk in circles, unable to pick up clues that once had guided him. He tapped through a room with his guide stick, no longer able to get his bearings. He once walked out of the house and into the street, not realizing that he was outside. A neighbor brought him home. Another time in the middle of the night he put water on to boil for tea and forgot about it, sending smoke through the kitchen. Luckily the smoke detector went off, alerting the sleeping household.

Harriet, more than anyone, could recognize and handle the gradual stages of decline.

Eventually, we all agreed to hire a person to stay with him a few hours a day. Millie came in the morning, helped with lunch, and talked to him. She guided him around the house to prevent his becoming tired or frustrated with fruitless searches.

Harriet told Marcia and me that the time would come when my father would require more supervision and attention than she could give at home, even with extra help. No one could have made a better home for my father. Only she knew how much to do for him and how much to let him do. Only she could say "No" to him because she was as strong-willed as he. He was demanding, but she could stand up to him. They argued, but she could deal with it. She and Bob, Randy, and Gail did for him what his other daughters and their families were not able to do. Harriet and her family had made a happy home for him for fifteen years. Now he would need more care than she could give. We would have to consider a nursing home

"I can't do it anymore" she said one day. "His safety and ours is at stake."

I could not accept the idea of a nursing home. I told myself that perhaps my father would stop this decline, that we would find another solution. Maybe if I helped Harriet more or if he could stay with me from time to time he would not need to go. I had talked it over with Dan who felt it was not a good idea for my father to stay at our house.

"We aren't set up the way Harriet is," Dan said. "He'll find it impossible to get around."

But I was determined to try to take care of my father, and Dan saw he could not change my mind.

"Let me take him to my house," I told Harriet. "Just for the weekend to start."

Harriet looked at me coldly. "Do you think you can take better care of him than I can?"

"Not better, Harriet. I need to try to keep him out of a nursing home. Maybe we can work it out if he comes to me."

"All right, do as you wish," she said as she turned away from me.

My father came to our house on Friday afternoon well before sundown. I arranged a bed on the sofa in our family room. I rigged up a rope from the family room to the bathroom to guide him—a distance of about ten or fifteen feet through the kitchen and around a corner. I put a monitor in the family room next to the sofa. It was the same one I had used when my children were little. It picked up every little sound and sigh.

During that night my father was up often to go to the bathroom. I could hear that even with the rope he was having trouble finding his way. I came down to help him. I had no sleep that night. Early Saturday, I made a cold breakfast for him because he was observant of the Sabbath laws which forbade turning on the stove. During the day I tried to read to him and help him in any way I could. Again I was up all Saturday night. By Sunday I was so tired because of two successive nights without sleep that I felt ill. I was overcome by the responsibility of caring for him. I was tense and anxious about what to do. When I brought my father back to Harriet's house, I knew I could not watch over him. Harriet said nothing to me.

My sisters and I called a family meeting to let everyone know what was happening. When our children and grandchildren all assembled, Harriet discussed the prospect of a nursing home. Everyone knew this option would not have been raised if there had been an alternative. They all knew that my father had become frail and forgetful. Each of them pledged to do whatever necessary to make things easier.

It was still hard for me to accept. At night in bed I cried. During my waking hours I would find tears rolling down my cheeks as I drove the car, as I shopped, as I sat and read.

"If you can't handle this," Harriet said, "get some professional help."

It seemed no one understood my grief. I didn't understand it myself. Was it that I defined myself as my father's daughter? Whenever I would meet longtime residents of Rochester I introduced myself and added, "I'm Sam Schafer's daughter." That was enough to gain recognition, acceptance, and respect. I had worked with him closely on all his projects, all his entrepreneurial efforts. We had shared the same goals of making a success of his ventures. Long before that, my sisters and I had worked in the store. Yet it was more than sharing a working life that had been so much a part of me.

"Daughters," I remember reading, "reflect the image their fathers give them." My father believed I could do anything he asked of me. I had pushed myself to do whatever he requested. I accomplished tasks that I had not believed I could do. I handled problems I never knew I could solve. I conquered fears I didn't know I could overcome.

I was losing my father to a nursing home—a place that I associated with death. I could not come to terms with that. My sisters and I made an appointment to meet the staff from the Jewish Home, where we took a tour and asked questions. I could not stop my tears. I just listened. My father was put on a waiting list. I sought professional help for myself.

We then had the delicate task of talking to my father about his entering the Jewish Home. Harriet, Marcia, and I sat with him and told him how we feared for his safety because he could not find his way around anymore.

"You shouldn't worry about me," he said. "I can find my way very good."

"No, Father, you're really getting lost a lot. That's why you get so tired sometimes," Marcia answered. "You could easily fall and get hurt when you get so tired."

Eventually he said he would try the Home. He would give it six months to see how it went. A heaviness fell upon me, an even greater oppressiveness than before. I shed more tears. Would I never stop? My sisters and I could not help each other. Here we were, trying to deal with the very same problem, and we could not bring comfort to each other, we who had always shared and helped each other before. It was only much later that I understood what was happening. We were each too involved in coping with our own feelings of guilt and sadness. It was the guilt that made it so difficult to reach out to one another. No one could help me, and I could not bring myself to offer solace to my sisters.

CHAPTER THIRTY-NINE

Stella Solaris

The nursing-home people told us they would call as soon as a room became available. It might take a few days or weeks or even months.

Meanwhile, my father started talking about taking another trip. "What a good idea," I said.

We had never taken so many consecutive trips. It was late winter of 1987, and I knew I could put a trip together for that summer, but Harriet and I began to argue immediately.

"He is too weak to go on a trip," Harriet said.

"It will lift his spirits and give him a boost," I answered.

"He hasn't got the strength for a long plane ride," Harriet countered.

"I'll find a short one."

"He needs attention and help all the time," she added.

"Everyone will help him in every way. We're all willing to do more, and I will stay with him if the others are busy."

Harriet was upset and anxious. "For whose benefit is this trip, yours or Father's?" she asked me. "He is too weak to enjoy it. Do you want this trip so badly that you are willing to jeopardize his health?"

I flinched as though she had struck me, and fell silent. Was I selfish—thinking of the chance to see another part of the world? Was I refusing to face my father's declining health and energy? Was I denying the knowledge that he was in the early stages of Alzheimer's disease? I did not think so. I was facing reality, and I thought I understood my motivation.

"I want another trip for us before he goes into the Home," I answered. "He loves all of the family being together. He's told me that before. He said, 'I can't see what we're doing, but I feel good when we are all on a trip together.' It means so much to him, and I think I can find a suitable trip that won't tire him. It will give all of us one last chance to share an adventure together. I want one more trip for him and for us."

Harriet was unmoved. "We must call a family meeting," she said. " Everyone needs to know how much help he will require. We have to make sure everybody knows ahead of time what's involved."

We assembled at Harriet's house. My father was already in bed. His hearing was so bad that we were sure he wouldn't hear us. Harriet told the group our concerns, and I explained that I was willing to look for a trip that would be short, easy, and enjoyable for everybody. The consensus pointed to a tentative agreement to go on a trip if I could find a suitable one.

I found a five-day cruise to Bermuda leaving from New York City on July 2, 1987. My father could sit through a one-hour plane ride to New York without discomfort. There would be no changing of planes, no hurried layovers, or sitting around an airport waiting.

We had coped with all kinds of plane connections in the past, and my father handled them. Once, years earlier, when all of us had been bumped from a scheduled flight, my father complained loudly to the hapless people behind the counter. The rest of us accepted the change in our flight without complaint. My father was impatient. At first he had not understood that we had been bumped. "Why are we standing around?" he had asked. "Let's keep moving."

Marcia explained that we had been taken off the scheduled flight and must wait for the next one.

"Take me to someone. I want to talk to a person in charge," he commanded. I took him to the desk. He was told we all would have to wait an hour for the next flight. "I don't want to wait for the next flight. I'm old and blind, and I want to get on the plane now, the way we're supposed to. I want to see the big boss around here," he had demanded.

I had taken him aside. "Father, you are talking to the big boss. It won't hurt us to wait an hour for the next flight. Don't put on this 'I'm old and blind' bit. He can see you're in better shape than most of us, even though you're blind. Stop getting all worked up."

He had muttered to himself and remained disgruntled. In a way, he seemed to relish these skirmishes with the hierarchy. Certainly he had been able to handle all the problems that had come up and was even willing to argue for us. Now it was different. He had become so frail.

I met with the travel agent and reviewed the details with her. We called another family meeting to explain the Bermuda trip and get everyone's opinion. Everyone voted to go. Fourteen of us began our preparations.

In June Harriet received a call from the Jewish Home. A place was available for my father the first week of July. We were not quite sure what to do. Harriet suggested that my father enter the Home the day after we returned from our trip. She told us that after the vacation he would have to get used to her house all over again.

"He can use his energy getting used to the Home. It will be easier for him than being transplanted again a few days later," she told us. It made sense to us. We told him, but planning the trip was foremost in his mind. It didn't seem to matter to him when he went into the Home.

A few days before we left Harriet showed me a chart she had made with everyone's name down one side and time slots across the top.

"What's this all about?" I asked her.

"It's a chart that everyone can fill in, so we make sure Father has someone to care for him at all times, and we can be sure that everyone is doing enough."

"Harriet, it's out of the question. How can anyone know before we're on the ship what he's going to want to do at a certain time? We have to do things the way we always do—in a natural way. We've had mini-meetings during our past trips to plan a day or two ahead. We haven't had any problems before, and we won't now."

We argued about this time sheet idea, but in the end it quietly died, and nothing more was said. We left as we always had, full of excitement and anticipation. This time, however, we knew it would be our last, and there was an overlay of sadness for us that never really left me. It was like mist engulfing us. Every minute was charged with special emotion. Our return would herald a new time in my father's life and ours—another transformation.

The trip to New York was uneventful. The *Stella Solaris,* an old refurbished ship, awaited us at the port. We settled in and immediately took my father through the usual orientation of his stateroom so he could find his way to the bathroom. The rooms were small, so it was hard to get lost, but either Randy or Paul, his roommates, were ready and willing to assist him.

On our previous cruise we had left the country from Florida. The southern waters had been calm. The northern Atlantic was rougher, and after a few hours a number of passengers felt sick, including several from our group. The ship tilted noticeably. My father and I took a short walk on deck and managed very well. I told him I was proud that we two were seaworthy, and we expressed sympathy for those who were beginning to feel poorly. Still, most of us enjoyed the evening's entertainment, although my father stayed in his room and went to bed.

The next morning I came down to breakfast to join my father and Harriet. They were early risers. I, too, liked getting up early on a trip.

As I slid into a chair across from them, Harriet asked, "Why are you here? You don't have to get up early to help me. I don't need any help now."

"I want to be here. I thought it would be nice if I joined you," I told her, surprised at her remarks.

Was she still angry about that chart with the time lines? We argued over who should go to breakfast and how many should go to breakfast.

"Why not let anyone who wants to get up early just be there? Why dictate breakfast?" I raised my voice, although I was not yet shouting. My father, who seemed deafer each day, did not appear to take notice of our heated exchange. This was the first of our arguments, but not the last. We bickered often, over matters that I no longer remember. Finally Marcia, our big sister, told us to quit acting like children and shape up. We each promised to control ourselves and act in a manner befitting intelligent adults. Long afterward, I looked back and tried to figure out why Harriet and I so often argued on this trip. I think we were both angry, not with each other perhaps, but at the way time changes all of us. Now our father was old and weak and often confused. How could such drastic changes take place and why? Certainly it shouldn't have happened to him—his blindness was enough of a misfortune, one that he had struggled with for many years. We could more easily accept his declining strength than the loss of his memory and sharpness of wit. The tension between us did not disappear, but we both remembered our promise to Marcia.

Many of our group wore patches behind their ears to control seasickness. Both Harriet and Bob felt the rolling of the ship, as well as Dan and Judy. Maureen felt it more than anyone. I did not mind the motion, although eating a meal was hard when the dishes and silverware clattered back and forth across the table. Our days at sea were difficult until we sailed into calmer waters. The night before we reached Bermuda we had a family meeting. Having pushed for the trip, and having promised at the outset that I would step in if everyone wanted to go ashore, Dan and I elected to stay on board with my father while the rest went to Hamilton, our only stop before returning to New York.

After waving good by to the family as they departed on the small boat that took them to shore, the three of us walked the deck and talked to the very few people who remained aboard. We enjoyed the quiet of the dining room at lunch. Of course, we had the undivided attention of the crew. In the late afternoon Maureen returned on the second last boat in. It would return to Hamilton one more time for an hour.

"Aunt Ruth and Uncle Dan, why don't you go into Hamilton on the last boat out? You'll have an hour to walk around. Grandpa and I will have some time together."

Maureen was a lot like her mother, vivacious and fun, thoughtful and generous. My father took great pleasure in her company. Dan and I quickly agreed to go and scrambled to get aboard the last tender. In a short time we were strolling through the palm-lined streets of Hamilton, looking at the people, the pastel colored houses and stores. I loved the scene around us, so colorful and exotic, and I was grateful that we had received the gift of an hour in Bermuda.

I spent the last two days at sea trying to keep cheerful, but I kept remembering that this was our last trip, and my father was going into a nursing home the day after our return. One evening I stopped into his stateroom to visit. We chatted awhile, and then he left his chair briefly to go to the bathroom, not more than a few feet away. Returning, he walked back to his chair slowly and with great effort. I saw the strain of concentration on his face. I witnessed his struggle to keep moving, to find the chair.

When he finally sat down he said, "I'm getting around pretty good. Don't you think so?"

"You're getting around wonderfully well. I think you're doing great," I told him.

I could feel my eyes fill with tears. They rolled down my face, but there was no need to brush them away. I was close to tears often—when I saw the grandchildren helping him at lunch, when I watched them walk with him on the deck, matching their steps to his slow and halting ones. When we all sat and talked together at dinner, I felt the poignant sense that such times would be forever gone.

I reminded myself that my father had long ago left his home in Europe and set out alone for an unknown destination. He had built a new life in America. He established a business, and reared a family. When he had been blinded, he began a new life living in his daughter's home, while retaining the role of patriarch for his family. When my mother died, and later Esther, he had shown us how to live with grief.

He had fashioned a way of living that was as productive and happy as he could make it. Now he would once more be thrust into a new life, in a different place. If the past was any indication of the future, I knew he would wrest from his circumstances whatever would bring pleasure and productivity. He would accept life at whatever terms were presented. I wept for him and for us as I thought of all we each had to learn to accept.

CHAPTER FORTY

Life in the Nursing Home

It was a bright and sunny day that Marcia, Harriet, and I brought my father into the nursing home. One of us helped my father while the others carted boxes of his possessions up to his room. We made several trips to the car, and I saw that Harriet and Marcia were upset, their faces tense. They both found it hard to control their tears. I was dry-eyed. I had cried myself out. Besides there was work to be done. I wanted to get my father settled in his room. This was no time for crying. I did not offer any words of comfort. I could only say to myself, "Now they understand how I felt. Now they actually know how hard this is."

I was still resentful that there had seemed to be so little sympathy for me when the nursing home decision had been made. It would take time for each of us to come to terms with our feelings. That day we still couldn't sort out our emotions. When Harriet asked if I would cooperate in making out a schedule of visiting our father I said no. I did not want to take turns on a prearranged basis. I wanted to visit him whenever I wished, and I could not make plans that would fit into a schedule. Perhaps Harriet thought I was unreasonable, but she did not press the matter, and the idea was dropped.

When we brought our father to his room that first day, I swept my eyes over the furniture. "Is the room nice?" my father asked as we got him seated in a chair.

"It's very nice," Harriet said. "It's a pretty-good-sized room. There's a window that lets in light and air. The bathroom's across from your side. You've got a roommate on the other side of the room."

His roommate lay in bed, oblivious of all us newcomers. His name, according to the label at the entrance to the room, was Dr. Golden. Next to Dr Golden sat his sister. Her skin was wrinkled, but heavily powdered with two bright spots of red on each cheek. She wore dark magenta lipstick. Her bright-orange hair stood out from her head in wild disarray. We found out later that she and her brother had shared a house all their lives, neither one having married.

His debilitating condition forced him into the nursing home several months earlier. It was the first time they had been separated. She glared at us, probably not happy with her brother's new roommate who came equipped with an entourage. We all introduced ourselves to Miss Golden, but she only nodded her head and said nothing.

Marcia began helping our father orient himself. She tried to show him how to get to the bathroom on the opposite side of the room. He was having trouble figuring it out.

"He needs to have his bed on the other side of the room," Harriet said. "The wall would guide him to the bathroom." Not wishing to tire him, Marcia stopped the orientation lesson. Harriet suggested that for now he ask the nurse for help if he needed to go to the bathroom.

"We must establish a presence here," I said. "The staff needs to know that Father has an involved family who will ask questions. That will get him more attention." We all agreed to make ourselves as visible as possible.

During the summer my sisters and I stopped into the home often. Harriet went twice a day the first week to help him during the transition. Marcia went as often as she could, and so did the grandsons. My father was always happy to talk to them. Paul, whose schedule was erratic, sometimes stopped by late at night, bringing with him my father's favorite hard candy. Whatever the hour, my father was pleased to see him. Maureen brought him one of his favorite treats—vanilla milkshakes. That summer I came often and went for walks with him. We usually ended our excursion at the café on the first floor where we sat and talked. Here, residents could have a beverage, ice cream, or fruit, as well as some other light snacks. Sometimes a long-ago-customer from the fish market joined us at our table. I remembered many of them. Forty or fifty years earlier they had been vibrant and strong, busy running their households, asking for the freshest fish, admonishing my father for not cleaning the fish enough, buying big orders for the holidays. Now they, too, were residents of the nursing home, frail and infirm.

"Of course I remember you, Mrs. Silver," I answered the inevitable question. "You were a very good customer. Oh, hello, Mrs. Goldenberg, how nice to see you. How could I forget you?" It was a mini -Joseph Avenue there in the café. Some of my father's former customers could not carry on a conversation with him because he was so hard of hearing. They did not have the strength to talk loudly enough, but when I was there we could carry on a three-way discussion. When any of the family talked to him in his room with the door shut, we could be heard in the hall. It was hard to talk about anything private because he couldn't hear us unless we shouted at him.

My father's roommate remained silent and still. Every time I saw him, he was lying in his bed motionless. Harriet reiterated that my father could not be as independent as possible as long as he needed assistance to the bathroom. He was annoyed at having to wait for a nurse to come to his aid. When Harriet told the nurse my father's bed should be on the other of the room, she agreed and told us to ask Dr. Golden's sister if we could change sides.

"May my father switch sides with your brother? The nurse will be glad to wheel your brother's bed to my father's side." Harriet smiled pleasantly at Miss Golden as she spoke to her.

The sister looked at Harriet and shook her head. "No, my brother can't change sides."

I thought we were not being clear. Perhaps she didn't understand the situation.

I restated our request. "My father is blind. If he were on the same side as the bathroom he could get out of bed, feel the wall and follow it to the bathroom without assistance. He wouldn't have to wait for someone to help him. Your brother does not get out of bed. It would mean a great deal to my father, and it doesn't seem that it would matter to your brother."

"No, I don't want him to change sides," she said.

The nurse did not want to press the issue. She told us she would look for another room for my father. We hoped for a private room, but we knew they were scarce. Several weeks later the nurse told us about a room that she was sure my father would like. His bed would be on the side with the bathroom. Moving day involved a little scurrying about with armfuls of clothes, pictures we had brought, his guide stick, talking clock, and a few other items.

"Is this a private room?" my father asked as we brought him into his new room.

"No," answered Harriet. "You have a roommate. His name is Lewis. He and his wife are waiting to be introduced to you. Thus began our friendship with Lewis's wife, Evelyn, a charming person who helped my father when one of us wasn't there, who gave us hints and clues about the staff and who proved to be a good friend. She came every day to sit with her husband, wheel him about, and make sure that he was comfortable and that his needs were met. Lewis was relatively young, but he lay in bed most of the time, incapacitated by Parkinson's Disease.

I went back to work when the fall term at school started. One of us stopped to see my father every day. I helped him with dinner, cutting up his food, explaining what was on his plate. He was capable of feeding himself. Besides visiting him, Harriet was also in touch with the doctor. She met with the dietitian several times to see if my father could receive meals he liked. My father took advantage of the various activities offered at the home. He went to a crafts class and made fuzzy little bears for the grandchildren.

"Do you need pot holders?" he asked everyone. He made them for the gift shop. All of us bought woven pot holders. He went to afternoon prayer services every day. Paul made it a point to go with him. If he couldn't, I took him or someone else in the family did. If no family member was available, an aide or a volunteer accompanied him. He knew the prayers by heart.

Sometimes we were all able to go out together for ice cream. We celebrated Dan's birthday at a restaurant Maureen managed—a kosher restaurant. He enjoyed our celebrations. Sometimes he came to each of our houses for dinner. We tried to cook only his favorite foods on those occasions.

He was doing well, and we felt good. We settled into a pattern that included the nursing home as a part of our lives.

It was almost two years before we had to change the pattern. He started to slow down even more. "I'm tired. I want to lay down," he said when he came to Harriet's house for a birthday party. If he visited Marcia or me he wanted to lie down and was not interested in eating or talking to anyone. Even his getting in or out of a car was hard.

It became too difficult for him to go anywhere outside the nursing home.

"Let's make a birthday party for him right here at the Home. The cafeteria people will help us," Paul suggested. The celebration was a big success, and for a while we held little parties in the cafeteria. When the Home made a Friday night dinner for the residents and their families we all went.

Once, when Harriet came to visit him, there were plumbing tools in a corner of the room and a plumber in the bathroom.

"Your father dropped his false teeth down the toilet." Evelyn, said. "It's caused quite a problem, but the toilet will be working before anyone has to use it."

I came upon the scene when everything was back to normal. "What happened to Father's teeth?" I asked Harriet. "He can't be without his teeth."

"Oh, they're fine," Harriet answered. "Father, why don't you smile for Ruth. See, there's no damage." The plumber returned a few weeks later when my father dropped his hearing aid down the toilet, and again when he dropped his teeth down for the second time.

My father continued to find it difficult to get around and find his way. One day when Evelyn had wheeled Lewis out of the room, my father returned from the bathroom and climbed into Lewis's bed to rest. The nurse found him and helped him to his own bed. Another time my father accidentally climbed into Lewis's bed when Lewis was in it. Lewis was too weak to protest. My father, trying to get comfortable in Lewis's bed, jostled the feeding tube that was connected to Lewis. He might have actually disconnected it. Evelyn, long-suffering and kind, finally felt compelled to say that my father was a health hazard to Lewis.

"Maybe we can put in for a private room for your father," the nurse said.

CHAPTER FORTY-ONE

Day and Night in
the Nursing Home

"Will you call the police? I need to report some serious problems here." said Ethel, her wrinkled face full of distress. She usually asked me to find a fireman or a policeman.

"I'll talk to someone on my way down," I told her. The large day room was bright from the sunlight pouring through the windows that lined one wall. A dozen residents or more sat around the room in various degrees of wakefulness. Although it was only mid afternoon several people sat with eyes closed and head bowed. Anna, who usually complained a great deal, was sitting quietly hugging three teddy bears.

In a corner an unfamiliar face was scrunched up ready to cry. The face was small and birdlike, but the sound from the small mouth was loud. "I want my mother. Where are you, Mother? Please come." The voice grew louder.

I walked through the room toward my father. Mary-Jane, a mean-tempered octogenarian, blocked my way. "Someone took my treat. I paid a lot of money for my treat—fourteen dollars. I worked very hard to make fourteen dollars, and so did my father."

"I'm sorry to hear someone took it," I said trying to placate her. "Wait a second. Here's a treat with your name on it."

From a table I picked up a cellophane-wrapped cookie with her name printed on a label across it.

"No, it's not. Mine is fourteen dollars." She wandered away toward the piano. A crone-like figure was already seated there, pounding erratically.

Above the noise, I imagined the room hummed with the restless, fluttering spirits of lost people trapped in old bodies. Did they have vague, elusive intimations of youth and health and vitality from a long-ago past?

My father sat by himself in a wheelchair. "Hi, Father. I'm here to see how you're doing today." I took his hand. He circled my wrist with his thumb and third finger.

"Rootie, you're too thin," he said, smiling toward the sound of my voice. "Are you eating enough?"

" Of course I am. C'mon, Father. Let me wheel you into the hall. There's no one out there."

"Don't bother. It's nice and quiet in here," he answered. I kept forgetting how hard of hearing he was.

A few nights later I met my nephew, Paul, at the nursing home. It was after the usual visiting time, but Paul often worked late and came when he could. The day room was empty and dark, chairs neatly tucked into the tables. I looked in. The room was silent. In his bedroom, my father lay awake, already greeting Paul.

"It's good to hear you. Sit down and relax. It's nice and quiet in here." They talked together. When I left it was almost eleven, but they were still deep in their conversation.

Such conversations were soon to become less frequent. He talked less and less. Although he answered questions, it was usually with a monosyllable or an, "I don't know." He was drifting away. His awareness of us and his pleasure in talking to friends and family were slowly disappearing. More and more I wondered if he knew anyone. It was as though we were on the shore, watching as he was carried further away from us by a relentless tide. There was nothing we could do.

CHAPTER FORTY-TWO

The Ending

My father stopped going to prayer service. Paul had taken him most often and stayed throughout the service. He helped him rise at the appropriate time and told him when to sit down. He whispered what was happening and tried to remind my father of parts of the service he thought my father might say with him. My father could not remember any of it. Even the words he had recited from earliest childhood were lost.

Then he began to disrupt the prayer service. "I want some ginger ale," or "I want to lay down." One of the worshippers told Paul that it was too distracting with my father there. Although Paul stopped taking him, Paul continued to go to services. Alone.

Does he know me today? I wondered as I entered the nursing home. I often came at dinner time. So many of the residents had trouble handling utensils that the aides were busy going from person to person, spoon feeding each one. They told me they were glad that I was there to help him. I explained what was on his plate, I cut up the food for him, and I brought him more ginger ale when he called out, "Get me some ginger ale." All of us saw the changes that were transforming him from the gregarious person we knew into a withdrawn stranger. He spoke to us without the typical warmth and enthusiasm that had once been part of him. When I left him each evening he sometimes, but not often, said,

"Goodbye." I tried not to think of what was happening to him—it caused too much pain.

I can't remember how his craving for ginger ale began. He started by asking for a glass, then two glasses. The aides told me he asked for some all through the day. I sometimes refilled his glass three or four times. "Father, you just had a lot of ginger ale. Did you forget?" I asked.

I told him he was probably drinking too much, but he kept repeating loudly, "Get me ginger ale."

I'd run to the refrigerator on his floor to refill his glass. A few times his floor ran out of ginger ale, probably because he used it up. I ran from floor to floor searching in each wing's refrigerator for a bottle.

"How come you're taking our ginger ale?" an aide sometimes asked as I rushed away.

"I'll return a bottle when the next shipment comes in up on the sixth floor." I answered.

During his last two years he experienced erratic mood changes. For a period of time he began to use his guide stick to swing wildly at people near him. He wielded the stick to hit the aides or residents. Everyone was very careful to stay clear of him. The nurse took away his guide stick.

"I need my guide stick," he yelled.

I tried to reason with him. "Father, you don't walk around very much. Whenever you take a walk with me I'll get your guide stick for you. When you need it you'll have it." Sometimes he calmed down.

Eventually his "wild phase" passed. After that period he sat in his wheelchair not moving or talking much. He didn't bother to wear his dark glasses. He had always insisted on wearing them. They had been essential to his wardrobe. I thought they added a certain dash to his appearance. He used to take them off at night, placing them on his night stand so he could reach them first thing in the morning. He never saw how his "eyes" looked, but he had believed that they might offend people. Actually, his eyelids were not fully open, and his appearance was marred by the injury.

He lost interest in the world around him, and spent more and more time in bed, saying, "I'm tired." I thought of all the effort it had taken him to be involved in the world, to take interest in all of us, to keep going despite the tremendous toll on his aging body. My sisters and I felt that he had used up almost all his strength.

Sometimes he was more alert than others, and more responsive to questions. At those times it was almost as though a window in his mind opened, letting in thoughts and ideas. He could converse a little. That rarely happened, but no matter whether he was alert or withdrawn we all kept coming to see him. From time to time he would have a serious health problem. Harriet was adamant that she must be notified in advance about what steps or procedures were going to be used. She was a health professional who could talk to the doctors with knowledge and authority about his condition and treatments. He came through a few bouts of pneumonia, prostate trouble, various infections, and the flu.

One time I came to his room and found him in his bed, crying tearlessly. "What's wrong, Father?" I asked, alarmed. "Does something hurt you?" I had not seen him overcome with emotion like this in a long time.

"I've lived too long," he sobbed. That window in his mind must have opened.

I took his hand. I didn't know what to say. "Father, we all want you to be here for us." I answered, "We love you and we need you." Should I have told him the truth, that I, too, grieved to see him helpless in a nursing home, cared for as one cares for a baby, a shell of the person he once was? I didn't know. I stopped talking and held his hand. In a little while the window closed anyway, but for a brief time he knew what was happening.

As his ninety-second birthday approached I thought we should have a little party on the sixth floor for him. "He won't know it's his birthday," Harriet said. "I doubt that he will recognize us."

She was probably right. For several months, I felt he had not recognized me at all, but that was not the whole point. "It may not matter to him," I said to Harriet, "but I think it matters to the rest of us. We can't know how many birthdays he has left. I think we should all get together to make a little celebration—to share our family love for him and each other, to acknowledge his years and his struggle."

Harriet understood. We had ice cream and cake—a cake big enough for every resident and aide on his wing. We brought it in before the shifts changed at three o'clock so that both shifts could enjoy it. Most of the children and grandchildren were there, and all of us talked and laughed together. My father, most of the time, seemed oblivious of us, but he did ask for ginger ale. I was glad we had the birthday party.

A number of times I met my nephew, Paul, when I went to see my father at dinner time. Together we wheeled my father out of the dining area and into the hallway. Paul liked the privacy of being alone in the hall without all the distracting behaviors of the dining room. Both of us helped him and made sure he had ginger ale.

"Grandpa," Paul asked, "Don't you remember how you told us to eat carrots? Here's some carrots for you right now. Isn't that great?" My father didn't answer. Paul guided my father's hand to the fork and helped him spear the piece of carrot. I wanted to actually feed my father by putting the fork to his lips, but Paul wouldn't let me.

"It's better for him to do as much as he can for himself. Don't do so much for him," he admonished me.

I tried to do as he suggested, but I wanted to make it easy for my father. I actually fed him so he didn't have to do anything but open his mouth. Whenever Paul saw me do that he shook his head at me and gently took the fork from my hand and put it into my father's. "Here, Grandpa," he'd say, "Here's your delicious green beans. Think of all the vitamins you're getting." My father would not answer.

One cold night in December I made myself go to the nursing home at dinner time, despite the blustery wind. Paul was already there in the hallway. "I just got here. It's a little wilder than usual in there tonight," he said as he motioned toward the dining room. "It's nice and quiet out here, isn't it, Grandpa? It's easier for us to talk." Paul often carried on a monologue with my father. How are you feeling, Grandpa?" he asked.

"Tip top," my father answered. "How are you, Pauli?"

I looked at Paul. He looked at me. We both looked at my father. His face was animated, alive looking. The smile of pleasure that he had worn when one of us was with him was on his face. He looked like himself. Gone was that vacant expression. I couldn't even remember when I had last seen him look so alive and natural.

"Father, I'm here, too. This is Ruth." I took his hand so he could feel my presence. He put his thumb and forefinger around my wrist.

"Rootie, you're still too thin. Look how skinny you are. I can put my fingers around your arm."

"Father, that's my wrist. I always had thin arms and legs, even when I was chubby."

"You have to eat more," my father laughingly said. I couldn't believe our conversation. Paul and I kept looking at each other. The window of his mind was wide open tonight.

"How's business, Paul?" my father asked. The two of them began talking about Paul's printing shop. I was silent, thinking how lucky Paul and I were to be with him at this rare and wonderful moment.

I told myself, *Ruth, he's here tonight. He's himself. Make sure to say the important things you never got to say to Mother. Tell him what you need to say to him.*

When there was a lull in his conversation with Paul, I put my hand on my father's, "Father, I love you."

"Thank you," he replied.

"You have always been a wonderful father. There's none better."

"Thank you very much."

"Look how much you accomplished, coming to this country with nothing except your tallis and tefillin. You should be very proud of all you were able to do."

"I always tried to do my best," he said modestly and smiled.

The three of us began talking together. Paul and I answered his questions about the weather and driving conditions. He didn't ask for ginger ale, but I got him a glass.

As he drank, Paul and I talked softly. "I'm worried," Paul said.

"About what?"

"I read or heard somewhere that a little while before a person dies, he's better than he's ever been in a long time."

"Your grandfather is tough," I said. "He's come through a lot, and he'll continue to come through for a long time. Don't worry any more."

My father died ten days later.

* * *

Paul was the last person to see my father alive. After the funeral I asked Paul to tell me what had happened their last time together.

"I went up to see him on Friday before sundown," he said. "Grandpa was lying on his side in bed. It was hard for him to breathe. It seemed as though his whole body rose and fell with every breath. I told him I was going to the prayer service downstairs, and I would be right back to help him with his dinner. He didn't say anything, but I knew he heard me. He turned over on his other side. As I went out the door, I stopped and looked back. I saw him put his head down carefully on his pillow. After the service—it took about forty-five minutes—I went back up to his room. He was just the way I last saw him. He hadn't moved, but I didn't hear or see him breathing. I went closer. He looked too quiet."

Paul knew something was wrong. He ran for the nurse, and she confirmed that my father was dead. What Paul had not known when he had gone to prayer service earlier and had looked back as he left my father's room, was that he was seeing my father positioning himself for his eternal sleep.

What, I wondered, had my father thought about before he died? Had his whole life flashed before him? Did he recall how he had taken big cans full of milk to the market town of Klimentov with the horses and wagon? Did he recall his mother's last embrace, his coming through Kesselgarden, his wedding, his treks to Cobbs Hill with his eight grandchildren? How many triumphs and failures of our real estate adventures did he remember? Did he envision all of us trailing after him through the streets of Tel Aviv or Paris, London or Madrid as he called out, "Let's keep moving"? Did he remember how he listened as we described the Western Wall, the Tower of London, the Iolani Palace, the Prado, the lights shimmering on the Seine? Could he recall our parties for him at the Jewish Home?

And what of the grandchildren? What will they remember of our trips and our family dinners? They have seen us laugh and cry, fight and make up. They know their grandfather was often impatient, sometimes difficult, and usually stubborn, but they saw that he embodied the strength he urged them to have in their daily lives. They witnessed his determination to discover a way through disaster and despair, through the sorrow of loss and the pain of grief.

"I'm a mechanical man," he once said to his grandson, David. "I have fake eyes, false teeth, a pacemaker, and I wear a hearing aid. I'm not a real man."

"Those things don't make a real person," David replied. "You care about us. You care about people, and you live every minute of your life. That makes you real." David, like the other grandchildren, knew the real Sam Schafer, had talked, laughed, and worked with him.

But what of the grandchildren's children? From their different time and place in the universe, will they come to understand this one thing— that the terrible accidents of life, the weight of history cannot crush someone who, like my father, willed himself to toast life over and over?

"L'chaim," he'd say, as he held up his glass, turned to us and repeated his favorite adage, "Let's keep moving."

EPILOGUE

The story is over. My father has been dead for years. I wrote of the lessons he tried to teach us. I told about what we had learned from his life and how he lived it. But it is now that I feel the power of his influence. Now, when my own daughter, Judy, lies dead, taken by cancer at the age of 45, that I appreciate his extraordinary strength.

When Esther, my sister, died at the age of 44, I was sure my father's spirit would be broken. He was 78. In wonder I watched as he slowly pulled himself together, once again assumed the role of patriarch. I watched as he turned his attention to helping us overcome our own grief at Esther's death.

He showed us we could recover our enjoyment of living. Eventually we celebrated the holidays with laughter. We began traveling together again—not the same without Esther, but with gratitude for what we once had and what we still had.

My father's example of how to bear grief strengthens me. He did it all in the dark, reaching out to all of us and helping to remind us that much of our strength derives from family and friends.

My father's spirit speaks to me today. It is saying that the most important things in life are courage and love.

S. Moldavskaya